Virtual Clinical Excursions—Obstetrics-P

for

Leifer:
Introduction to Maternity and Pediatric Nursing,
7th Edition

Virtual Clinical Excursions—Obstetrics-Pediatrics

for

Leifer:
Introduction to Maternity and Pediatric Nursing, 7th Edition

prepared by

Kim D. Cooper, RN, MSN
Dean, School of Nursing
Ivy Tech Community College
Terre Haute, Indiana

software developed by
Wolfsong Informatics, LLC
Tucson, Arizona

ELSEVIER
SAUNDERS

ELSEVIER
SAUNDERS

3251 Riverport Lane
Maryland Heights, Missouri 63043

VIRTUAL CLINICAL EXCURSIONS—OBSTETRICS-PEDIATRICS FOR
LEIFER: INTRODUCTION TO MATERNITY AND PEDIATRIC NURSING,
SEVENTH EDITION

ISBN: 978-0-323-32781-7

Copyright © 2015, 2011, 2007 by Saunders, an imprint of Elsevier Inc.

Notice

Knowledge and best practice in this field are constantly changing. As new research and experience broaden our understanding, changes in research methods, professional practices, or medical treatment may become necessary.

Practitioners and researchers must always rely on their own experience and knowledge in evaluating and using any information, methods, compounds, or experiments described herein. In using such information or methods they should be mindful of their own safety and the safety of others, including parties for whom they have a professional responsibility.

With respect to any drug or pharmaceutical products identified, readers are advised to check the most current information provided (i) on procedures featured or (ii) by the manufacturer of each product to be administered, to verify the recommended dose or formula, the method and duration of administration, and contraindications. It is the responsibility of practitioners, relying on their own experience and knowledge of their patients, to make diagnoses, to determine dosages and the best treatment for each individual patient, and to take all appropriate safety precautions.

To the fullest extent of the law, neither the Publisher nor the authors, contributors, or editors, assume any liability for any injury and/or damage to persons or property as a matter of products liability, negligence or otherwise, or from any use or operation of any methods, products, instructions, or ideas contained in the material herein.

ISBN: 978-0-323-32781-7

Printed in the United States of America

Last digit is the print number: 9 8 7 6 5 4 3

*Workbook
prepared by*

Kim D. Cooper, RN, MSN
Dean, School of Nursing
Ivy Tech Community College
Terre Haute, Indiana

*Previous edition
prepared by*

Kelly Ann Crum, RN, MSN
Chair, Department of Nursing
Associate Professor of Nursing
Maranatha Baptist Bible College
Watertown, Wisconsin

Betty W. Hamlisch, RN, MS Health Education
Professor of Nursing
Tompkins Cortland Community College
Dryden, New York

Textbook

Gloria Leifer, RN, MA, CNE
Professor, Obstetric and Pediatric Nursing
Riverside City College
Riverside, California

Table of Contents
Virtual Clinical Excursions Workbook

Getting Started

Lessons

Table of Contents
Leifer: Introduction to Maternity and Pediatric Nursing, 7th Edition

Unit Five—The Child Needing Nursing Care

Unit Six—The Changing Health Care Environment

Appendixes

GETTING SET UP WITH VCE ONLINE ————————————————

The product you have purchased is part of the Evolve Learning System. Please read the following information thoroughly to get started.

■ HOW TO ACCESS YOUR VCE RESOURCES ON EVOLVE

There are two ways to access your VCE Resources on Evolve:

1. If your instructor has enrolled you in your VCE Evolve Resources, you will receive an email with your registration details.

2. If your instructor has asked you to self-enroll in your VCE Evolve Resources, he or she will provide you with your Course ID (for example, 1479_jdoe73_0001). You will then need to follow the instructions at https://evolve.elsevier.com/cs/studentEnroll.html.

■ HOW TO ACCESS THE ONLINE VIRTUAL HOSPITAL

The online virtual hospital is available through the Evolve VCE Resources. There is no software to download or install: the online virtual hospital runs within your Internet browser, using a pop-up window.

■ TECHNICAL REQUIREMENTS

- Broadband connection (DSL or cable)
- 1024 x 768 screen resolution
- Mozilla Firefox 18.0, Internet Explorer 9.0, Google Chrome, or Safari 5 (or higher)
  Note: Pop-up blocking software/settings must be disabled.
- Adobe Acrobat Reader
- Additional technical requirements available at http://evolvesupport.elsevier.com

■ HOW TO ACCESS THE WORKBOOK

There are two ways to access the workbook portion of *Virtual Clinical Excursions:*

1. Print workbook
2. An electronic version of the workbook, available within the VCE Evolve Resources

■ TECHNICAL SUPPORT

Technical support for *Virtual Clinical Excursions* is available by visiting the Technical Support Center at http://evolvesupport.elsevier.com or by calling 1-800-222-9570 inside the United States and Canada.

Trademarks: Windows® and Macintosh® are registered trademarks.

A QUICK TOUR

Welcome to *Virtual Clinical Excursions—Obstetrics-Pediatrics*, a virtual hospital setting in which you can work with multiple complex patient simulations and also learn to access and evaluate the information resources that are essential for high-quality patient care. The virtual hospital, Pacific View Regional Hospital, has realistic architecture and access to patient rooms, a Nurses' Station, and a Medication Room.

■ BEFORE YOU START

Make sure you have your textbook nearby when you use *Virtual Clinical Excursions*. You will want to consult topic areas in your textbook frequently while working with the virtual hospital and workbook.

■ HOW TO SIGN IN

- Enter your name on the Student Nurse identification badge.
- Next, click the down arrow next to **Select Floor**. For this quick tour, choose **Obstetrics**.
- Now click the down arrow next to **Select Period of Care**. This drop-down menu gives you four periods of care from which to choose. In Periods of Care 1 through 3, you can actively engage in patient assessment, entry of data in the electronic patient record (EPR), and medication administration. Period of Care 4 presents the day in review. Highlight and click the appropriate period of care. (For this quick tour, choose **Period of Care 1: 0730-0815**.)
- Click **Go**. This takes you to the Patient List screen (see the *How to Select a Patient* section below). Note that the virtual time is provided in the box at the lower left corner of the screen (0730, since we chose Period of Care 1).

Note: If you choose to work during Period of Care 4: 1900-2000, the Patient List screen is skipped since you are not able to visit patients or administer medications during the shift. Instead, you are taken directly to the Nurses' Station, where the records of all the patients on the floor are available for your review.

■ **PATIENT LIST**

OBSTETRICS UNIT

Dorothy Grant (Room 201)
30-week intrauterine pregnancy—A 25-year-old multipara Caucasian female admitted with abdominal trauma following a domestic violence incident. Her complications include preterm labor and extensive social issues such as acquiring safe housing for her family upon discharge.

Stacey Crider (Room 202)
27-week intrauterine pregnancy—A 21-year-old primigravida Native American female admitted for intravenous tocolysis, bacterial vaginosis, and poorly controlled insulin-dependent gestational diabetes. Strained family relationships and social isolation complicate this patient's ability to comply with strict dietary requirements and prenatal care.

Kelly Brady (Room 203)
26-week intrauterine pregnancy—A 35-year-old primigravida Caucasian female urgently admitted for progressive symptoms of preeclampsia. A history of inadequate coping with major life stressors leave her at risk for a recurrence of depression as she faces a diagnosis of HELLP syndrome and the delivery of a severely premature infant.

Maggie Gardner (Room 204)
22-week intrauterine pregnancy—A 41-year-old multigravida African-American female admitted for a high-risk pregnancy evaluation and rule out diagnosis of systemic lupus erythematosus. Coping with chronic pain, fatigue, and a history of multiple miscarriages contribute to an anxiety disorder and the need for social service intervention.

Gabriela Valenzuela (Room 205)
34-week intrauterine pregnancy—A 21-year-old primigravida Hispanic female with a history of mitral valve prolapse admitted for uterine cramping and vaginal bleeding suggestive of placental abruption following an unrestrained motor vehicle accident. Her needs include staff support for an unprepared-for labor and possible preterm birth.

Laura Wilson (Room 206)
37-week intrauterine pregnancy—An 18-year-old primigravida Caucasian female urgently admitted after being found unconscious at home. Her complications include HIV-positive status and chronic polysubstance abuse. Unrealistic expectations of parenthood and living with a chronic illness combined with strained family relations prompt comprehensive social and psychiatric evaluations initiated on the day of simulation.

PEDIATRICS UNIT

George Gonzalez (Room 301)
Diabetic ketoacidosis—An 11-year-old Hispanic male admitted for stabilization of blood glucose level and diabetic re-education associated with his diagnosis of type 1 diabetes mellitus. This patient's poor compliance with insulin therapy and dietary regime have resulted in frequent and repeated hospital admissions for diabetic ketoacidosis.

Tommy Douglas (Room 302)
Traumatic brain injury—A 6-year-old Caucasian male transferred from the Pediatric Intensive Care Unit in preparation for organ donation. This patient is status post ventriculostomy with negative intracerebral blood flow and requires extensive hemodynamic monitoring and support, along with compassionate family care.

Carrie Richards (Room 303)
Bronchiolitis—A 3½-month-old African-American female admitted with respiratory distress due to respiratory syncytial virus, along with dehydration and an inadequate nutritional status. Parent education and support are among her primary needs.

Stephanie Brown (Room 304)
Meningitis—A 3-year-old African-American female with a history of spastic cerebral palsy admitted for intravenous antibiotic therapy, neurologic monitoring, and support for a diagnosis of acute meningitis. Maintenance of physical and occupational programs addressing her mobility limitations complicate her acute care stay.

Tiffany Sheldon (Room 305)
Anorexia nervosa—A 14-year-old Caucasian female admitted for dehydration, electrolyte imbalance, and malnutrition following a syncope episode at home. This patient has a history of eating disorders, which have resulted in multiple hospital admissions and strained family dynamics between mother and daughter.

■ HOW TO SELECT A PATIENT

- You can choose one or more patients to work with from the Patient List by checking the box to the left of the patient name(s). For this quick tour, select Dorothy Grant. (In order to receive a scorecard for a patient, the patient must be selected before proceeding to the Nurses' Station.)
- Click on **Get Report** to the right of the medical records number (MRN) to view a summary of the patient's care during the 12-hour period before your arrival on the unit.
- After reviewing the report, click on **Go to Nurses' Station** in the right lower corner to begin your care. (*Note:* If you have been assigned to care for multiple patients, you can click on **Return to Patient List** to select and review the report for each additional patient before going to the Nurses' Station.)

Note: Even though the Patient List is initially skipped when you sign in to work for Period of Care 4, you can still access this screen if you wish to review the shift report for any of the patients. To do so, simply click on **Patient List** near the top left corner of the Nurses' Station (or click on the clipboard to the left of the Kardex). Then click on **Get Report** for the patient(s) whose care you are reviewing. This may be done during any period of care.

Patient List

	Patient Name	Room	MRN	Clinical Report
☑	Dorothy Grant	201	1868096	Get Report
☐	Stacey Crider	202	1868065	Get Report
☐	Kelly Brady	203	1868073	Get Report
☐	Maggie Gardner	204	1868085	Get Report
☐	Gabriela Valenzuela	205	1868090	Get Report
☐	Laura Wilson	206	1868098	Get Report

Please select all the patients you will be caring for this period of care. Once you have exited the patient list, you will not be able to change your current selections or select new patients to care for.

0730   Go to Nurses' Station

■ **HOW TO FIND A PATIENT'S RECORDS**

NURSES' STATION

Within the Nurses' Station, you will see:

1. A clipboard that contains the patient list for that floor.
2. A chart rack with patient charts labeled by room number, a notebook labeled Kardex, and a notebook labeled MAR (Medication Administration Record).
3. A desktop computer with access to the Electronic Patient Record (EPR).
4. A tool bar across the top of the screen that can also be used to access the Patient List, EPR, Chart, MAR, and Kardex. This tool bar is also accessible from each patient's room.
5. A Drug Guide containing information about the medications you are able to administer to your patients.
6. A Laboratory Guide containing normal value ranges for all laboratory tests you may come across in the virtual patient hospital.
7. A tool bar across the bottom of the screen that can be used to access the Floor Map, patient rooms, Medication Room, and Drug Guide.

As you run your cursor over an item, it will be highlighted. To select, simply click on the item. As you use these resources, you will always be able to return to the Nurses' Station by clicking on the **Return to Nurses' Station** bar located in the right lower corner of your screen.

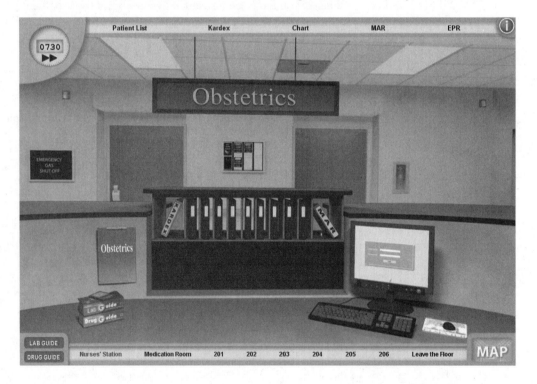

MEDICATION ADMINISTRATION RECORD (MAR)

The MAR icon located on the tool bar at the top of your screen accesses current 24-hour medications for each patient. Click on the icon and the MAR will open. (*Note:* You can also access the MAR by clicking on the MAR notebook on the far right side of the book rack in the center of the screen.) Within the MAR, tabs on the right side of the screen allow you to select patients by room number. Be careful to make sure you select the correct tab number for *your* patient rather than simply reading the first record that appears after the MAR opens. Each MAR sheet lists the following:

- Medications
- Route and dosage of each medication
- Times of administration of each medication

Note: The MAR changes each day. Expired MARs are stored in the patients' charts.

Pacific View Regional Hospital		MRN: 1868096	Room: 201	**201**
6475 E. Duke Avenue		Patient: Dorothy Grant		**202**
		Sex: Female	Age: 25	
		Physician: John Shelby, M.D.		**203**

Medication Administration Record
Wednesday

START	STOP	MEDICATION	0701-1900	1901-0700
Wed 0345		Lactated Ringer's 125 mL/hr IV continuous	1400	
Wed 0730	Wed 1930	Betamethasone 12 mg IM every 12 hours for 2 doses, dose #1	0730	1930
Wed 0730		Prenatal multivitamin 1 PO daily	0800	

ORD.	TTBG*.	STAT/PRE-OP/ONE TIME	TG**	INJECTION SITE CODE	
0730	today	Rho(D) Immune Globulin 1 vial (300 mcg) IM x 1		1. R Deltoid 2. L Deltoid 3. R Anterolateral Abdomen 4. L Anterolateral Abdomen 5. R Lateral Thigh	6. L Lateral Thigh 7. R Anterior Thigh 8. L Anterior Thigh 9. R Ventrogluteal 10. L Ventrogluteal

204
205
206

0732   Return to Nurses' Station

Charts

To access patient charts, either click on the **Chart** icon at the top of your screen or anywhere within the chart rack in the center of the Nurses' Station screen. When the close-up view appears, the individual charts are labeled by room number. To open a chart, click on the room number of the patient whose chart you wish to review. The patient's name and allergies will appear on the left side of the screen, along with a list of tabs on the right side of the screen, allowing you to view the following data:

- Allergies
- Physician's Orders
- Physician's Notes
- Nurse's Notes
- Laboratory Reports
- Diagnostic Reports
- Surgical Reports
- Consultations

- Patient Education
- History and Physical
- Nursing Admission
- Expired MARs
- Consents
- Mental Health
- Admissions
- Emergency Department

Information appears in real time. The entries are in reverse chronologic order, so use the down arrow at the right side of each chart page to scroll down to view previous entries. Flip from tab to tab to view multiple data fields or click on **Return to Nurses' Station** in the lower right corner of the screen to exit the chart.

Pacific View Regional Hospital **6475 E. Duke Avenue**	**MRN:** 1868096 **Room:** 201 **Patient:** Dorothy Grant **Sex:** Female **Age:** 25 **Physician:** John Shelby, M.D.	

Physician's Progress Notes

Day/Time	Notes	Signature
Wed 0730	25-year-old Caucasian female, G5, P3, AB 1, 30 weeks gestation, seen in ED for blunt abdominal trauma secondary to husband hitting and kicking abdomen of patient. Fundal height 29 cm. Ecchymosis and abrasions apparent on left lower abdomen and forearms. Remainder of physical examination WNL. OB ultrasound revealed normal fundal placement of placenta with no evidence of abruption. Fetus active with FHR in 130s. Admitted for observation. Mild contractions started approximately 2 hours after admission. Plan: 1. IV LR 500 mL bolus, then at 125 mL/hr. 2. Tocolysis if contractions continue. 3. Social services and Psychiatric consult. 4. Rho(D)Immune globulin for O negative blood type (patient missed her 28 week appointment and did not receive the Rho(D)Immune globulin at that time). 5. Betamethasone now and again in 12 hours if not delivered.	*Albert Seng, M.D.*

Allergies
Physician's Orders
Physician's Notes
Nurse's Notes
Laboratory Reports
Diagnostic Reports
Surgical Reports
Consultations
Patient Education
History and Physical
Nursing Admission
Expired MARs
Consents
Mental Health
Admissions
Emergency Department

0732

Return to Nurses' Station

ELECTRONIC PATIENT RECORD (EPR)

The EPR can be accessed from the computer in the Nurses' Station or from the EPR icon located in the tool bar at the top of your screen. To access a patient's EPR:

- Click on either the computer screen or the **EPR** icon.
- Your username and password are automatically filled in.
- Click on **Login** to enter the EPR.
- *Note:* Like the MAR, the EPR is arranged numerically. Thus when you enter, you are initially shown the records of the patient in the lowest room number on the floor. To view the correct data for *your* patient, remember to select the correct room number, using the drop-down menu for the Patient field at the top left corner of the screen.

The EPR used in Pacific View Regional Hospital represents a composite of commercial versions being used in hospitals. You can access the EPR:

- to review existing data for a patient (by room number).
- to enter data you collect while working with a patient.

The EPR is updated daily, so no matter what day or part of a shift you are working, there will be a current EPR with the patient's data from the past days of the current hospital stay. This type of simulated EPR allows you to examine how data for different attributes have changed over time, as well as to examine data for all of a patient's attributes at a particular time. The EPR is fully functional (as it is in a real-life hospital). You can enter such data as blood pressure, breath sounds, and certain treatments. The EPR will not, however, allow you to enter data for a previous time period. Use the arrows at the bottom of the screen to move forward and backward in time.

Patient: 201	Category: Vital Signs			0735	
Name: Dorothy Grant	**Wed 0700**	**Wed 0715**	**Wed 0733**	**Code Meanings**	
PAIN: LOCATION	A			A	Abdomen
PAIN: RATING	1-2			Ar	Arm
PAIN: CHARACTERISTICS	I			B	Back
PAIN: VOCAL CUES				C	Chest
PAIN: FACIAL CUES				Ft	Foot
PAIN: BODILY CUES				H	Head
PAIN: SYSTEM CUES				Hd	Hand
PAIN: FUNCTIONAL EFFECTS				L	Left
PAIN: PREDISPOSING FACTORS				Lg	Leg
PAIN: RELIEVING FACTORS				Lw	Lower
PCA				N	Neck
TEMPERATURE (F)	98.2			NN	See Nurses notes
TEMPERATURE (C)				OS	Operative site
MODE OF MEASUREMENT	O			Or	See Physicians orders
SYSTOLIC PRESSURE	126			PN	See Progress notes
DIASTOLIC PRESSURE	68			R	Right
BP MODE OF MEASUREMENT	NIBP			Up	Upper
HEART RATE	70				
RESPIRATORY RATE	18				
SpO2 (%)	96				
BLOOD GLUCOSE					
WEIGHT					
HEIGHT					

Return to Nurses' Station

At the top of the EPR screen, you can choose patients by their room numbers. In addition, you have access to 17 different categories of patient data. To change patients or data categories, click the down arrow to the right of the room number or category.

The categories of patient data in the EPR are as follows:

- Vital Signs
- Respiratory
- Cardiovascular
- Neurologic
- Gastrointestinal
- Excretory
- Musculoskeletal
- Integumentary
- Reproductive
- Psychosocial
- Wounds and Drains
- Activity
- Hygiene and Comfort
- Safety
- Nutrition
- IV
- Intake and Output

Remember, each hospital selects its own codes. The codes used in the EPR at Pacific View Regional Hospital may be different from ones you have seen in your clinical rotations. Take some time to acquaint yourself with the codes. Within the Vital Signs category, click on any item in the left column (e.g., Pain: Characteristics). In the far-right column, you will see a list of code meanings for the possible findings and/or descriptors for that assessment area.

You will use the codes to record the data you collect as you work with patients. Click on the box in the last time column to the right of any item and wait for the code meanings applicable to that entry to appear. Select the appropriate code to describe your assessment findings and type it in the box. (*Note:* If no cursor appears within the box, click on the box again until the blue shading disappears and the blinking cursor appears.) Once the data are typed in this box, they are entered into the patient's record for this period of care only.

To leave the EPR, click on **Exit EPR** in the bottom right corner of the screen.

■ **VISITING A PATIENT**

From the Nurses' Station, click on the room number of the patient you wish to visit (in the tool bar at the bottom of your screen). Once you are inside the room, you will see a still photo of your patient in the top left corner. To verify that this is the correct patient, click on the **Check Armband** icon to the right of the photo. The patient's identification data will appear. If you click on **Check Allergies** (the next icon to the right), a list of the patient's allergies (if any) will replace the photo.

Also located in the patient's room are multiple icons you can use to assess the patient or the patient's medications. A virtual clock is provided in the upper left corner of the room to monitor your progress in real time. (*Note:* The fast-forward icon within the virtual clock will advance the time by 2-minute intervals when clicked.)

- The tool bar across the top of the screen allows you to check the **Patient List**, access the **EPR** to check or enter data, and view the patient's **Chart**, **MAR**, or **Kardex**.

- The **Take Vital Signs** icon allows you to measure the patient's up-to-the-minute blood pressure, oxygen saturation, temperature, heart rate, respiratory rate, and pain level.

- Each time you enter a patient's room, you are given an Initial Observation report to review (in the text box under the patient's photo). These notes are provided to give you a "look" at the patient as if you had just stepped into the room. You can also click on the **Initial Observations** icon to return to this box from other views within the patient's room. To the right of this icon is **Clinical Alerts**, a resource that allows you to make decisions about priority medication interventions based on emerging data collected in real time. Check this screen throughout your period of care to avoid missing critical information related to recently ordered or STAT medications.

- Clicking on **Patient Care** opens up three specific learning environments within the patient room: **Physical Assessment**, **Nurse-Client Interactions**, and **Medication Administration**.

- To perform a **Physical Assessment**, choose a body area (such as **Head & Neck**) from the column of yellow buttons. This activates a list of system subcategories for that body area (e.g., see **Sensory**, **Neurologic**, etc. in the green boxes). After you select the system you wish to evaluate, a brief description of the assessment findings will appear in a box to the right. A still photo provides a "snapshot" of how an assessment of this area might be done or what the finding might look like. For every body area, you can also click on **Equipment** on the right side of the screen.

- To the right of the Physical Assessment icon is **Nurse-Client Interactions**. Clicking on this icon will reveal the times and titles of any videos available for viewing. (*Note:* If the video you wish to see is not listed, this means you have not yet reached the correct virtual time to view that video. Check the virtual clock; you may return to access the video once its designated time has occurred—as long as you do so within the same period of care. Or you can click on the fast-forward icon within the virtual clock to advance the time by 2-minute intervals. You will then need to click again on **Patient Care** and **Nurse-Client Interactions** to refresh the screen.) To view a listed video, click on the white arrow to the right of the video title. Use the control buttons below the video to start, stop, pause, rewind, or fast-forward the action or to mute the sound.

- **Medication Administration** is the pathway that allows you to review and administer medications to a patient after you have prepared them in the Medication Room. This process is also addressed further in the *How to Prepare Medications* section below and in *Medications* in **A Detailed Tour**. For additional hands-on practice, see *Reducing Medication Errors* below **A Quick Tour** and **A Detailed Tour** in your resources.

■ HOW TO CHANGE PATIENTS OR CHANGE PERIODS OF CARE

How to Change Patients or Periods of Care: To change patients, simply click on the new patient's room number. (You cannot receive a scorecard for a new patient, however, unless you have already selected that patient on the Patient List screen.) To change to a new period of care or to restart the virtual clock, click on **Leave the Floor** and then on **Restart the Program**.

Floor Menu

Look at your Preceptor's Evaluation.
Evaluations provide feedback on the work you completed during patient care. If you choose the Preceptor's Evaluation you will no longer be able to return to the floor.

Take a break.
Time will be stopped until you wish to return to the simulation.

Restart the program.
If you restart, all data from your work in the current Period of Care will be erased.

CREDITS **View Credits.**
Take a look at the list of professionals who took part in the creation of this software suite.

0743   Return to Nurses' Station

■ HOW TO PREPARE MEDICATIONS

From the Nurses' Station or the patient's room, you can access the Medication Room by clicking on the icon in the tool bar at the bottom of your screen to the left of the patient room numbers.

In the Medication Room you have access to the following (from left to right):

- A preparation area is located on the counter under the cabinets. To begin the medication preparation process, click on the tray on the counter or click on the **Preparation** icon at the top of the screen. The next screen leads you through a specific sequence (called the Preparation Wizard) to prepare medications one at a time for administration to a patient. However, no medication has been selected at this time. We will do this while working with a patient in **A Detailed Tour**. To exit this screen, click on **View Medication Room**.

- To the right of the cabinets (and above the refrigerator), IV storage bins are provided. Click on the bins themselves or on the **IV Storage** icon at the top of the screen. The bins are labeled **Microinfusion**, **Small Volume**, and **Large Volume**. Click on an individual bin to see a list of its contents. If you needed to prepare an IV medication at this time, you could click on the medication and its label would appear to the right under the patient's name. (*Note:* You can **Open** and **Close** any medication label by clicking the appropriate icon.) Next, you would click **Put Medication on Tray**. If you ever change your mind or decide that you have put the incorrect medication on the tray, you can reverse your actions by highlighting the medication on the tray and then clicking **Put Medication in Bin**. Click **Close Bin** in the right bottom corner to exit. **View Medication Room** brings you back to a full view of the entire room.

- A refrigerator is located under the IV storage bins to hold any medications that must be stored below room temperature. Click on the refrigerator door or on the **Refrigerator** icon at the top of the screen. Then click on the close-up view of the door to access the medications. When you are finished, click **Close Door** and then **View Medication Room**.

- To prepare controlled substances, click the **Automated System** icon at the top of the screen or click the computer monitor located to the right of the IV storage bins. A login screen will appear; your name and password are automatically filled in. Click **Login**. Select the patient for whom you wish to access medications; then select the correct medication drawer to open (they are stored alphabetically). Click **Open Drawer**, highlight the proper medication, and choose **Put Medication on Tray**. When you are finished, click **Close Drawer** and then **View Medication Room**.

- Next to the Automated System is a set of drawers identified by patient room number. To access these, click on the drawers or on the **Unit Dosage** icon at the top of the screen. This provides a close-up view of the drawers. To open a drawer, click on the room number of the patient you are working with. Next, click on the medication you would like to prepare for the patient, and a label will appear, listing the medication strength, units, and dosage per unit. To exit, click **Close Drawer**; then click **View Medication Room**.

At any time, you can learn about a medication you wish to prepare for a patient by clicking on the **Drug** icon in the bottom left corner of the medication room screen or by clicking the **Drug Guide** book on the counter to the right of the unit dosage drawers. The **Drug Guide** provides information about the medications commonly included in nursing drug handbooks. Nutritional supplements and maintenance intravenous fluid preparations are not included. Highlight a medication in the alphabetical list; relevant information about the drug will appear in the screen below. To exit, click **Return to Medication Room**.

To access the MAR from the Medication Room and to review the medications ordered for a patient, click on the **MAR** icon located in the tool bar at the top of your screen and then click on the correct tab for your patient's room number. You may also click the **Review MAR** icon in the tool bar at the bottom of your screen from inside each medication storage area.

After you have chosen and prepared medications, go to the patient's room to administer them by clicking on the room number in the bottom tool bar. Inside the patient's room, click **Patient Care** and then **Medication Administration** and follow the proper administration sequence.

■ PRECEPTOR'S EVALUATIONS

When you have finished a session, click on **Leave the Floor** to go to the Floor Menu. At this point, you can click on the top icon (**Look at Your Preceptor's Evaluation**) to receive a score-card that provides feedback on the work you completed during patient care.

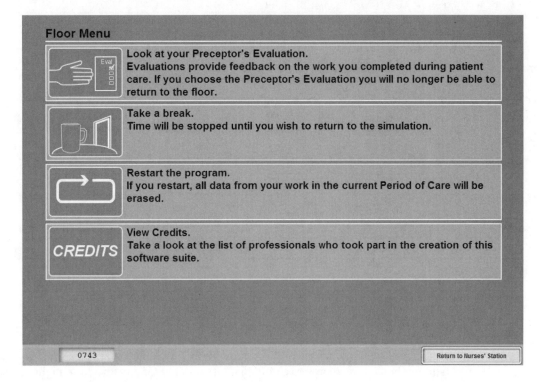

Evaluations are available for each patient you selected when you signed in for the current period of care. Click on the **Medication Scorecard** icon to see an example.

Medication Scorecard

Name:	Erin Taylor	Evaluation For: Dorothy Grant, Period of Care 1
Start Time:	0730	
End Time:	0744	

Instructions

Table A shows the medications that should have been administered to **Dorothy Grant** and also shows if you gave those medications as ordered during this period of care. Table B lists the medications that you administered incorrectly: **Wrong Dosage, Wrong Route/Method/Site, or Wrong Time**. Compare Tables A and B to see where you made errors. Table C lists how often you accessed patient's medical records, as well as listing the times that you checked critical patient information, such as; Arm Band, Allergy Band, Clinical Update, and Vital Signs. Table D lists all other medications administered to other patients during this period of care. Use the information in Table D to determine if you administered a medication to the wrong patient.

Table A: Medications that should have been administered to **Dorothy Grant** during this period of care.

Medication	Total Dosage	Route/Method/Site	Time	√ / X
Betamethasone	3 mL	Injection / Intramuscular / Any	0730-0815	√
Prenatal multivitamin	1 multivitamin	Oral / Any	0730-0815	√

√ = Correct   X = Incorrect

Table B: Erin Taylor, administered the following medications to **Dorothy Grant** incorrectly. Medications on this list were administered incorrectly, either by **Wrong Dosage, Wrong Route/Method/Site, or Wrong Time**.

Print		Return to Evaluations

The scorecard compares the medications you administered to a patient during a period of care with what should have been administered. Table A lists the correct medications. Table B lists any medications that were administered incorrectly.

Remember, not every medication listed on the MAR should necessarily be given. For example, a patient might have an allergy to a drug that was ordered, or a medication might have been improperly transcribed to the MAR. Predetermined medication "errors" embedded within the program challenge you to exercise critical thinking skills and professional judgment when deciding to administer a medication, just as you would in a real hospital. Use all your available resources, such as the patient's chart and the MAR, to make your decision.

Table C lists the resources that were available to assist you in medication administration. It also documents whether and when you accessed these resources. For example, did you check the patient armband or perform a check of vital signs? If so, when?

You can click **Print** to get a copy of this report if needed. When you have finished reviewing the scorecard, click **Return to Evaluations** and then **Return to Menu**.

■ FLOOR MAP

To get a general sense of your location within the hospital, you can click on the **Map** icon found in the lower right corner of most of the screens in the *Virtual Clinical Excursions—Obstetrics-Pediatrics* program. (*Note:* If you are following this quick tour step by step, you will need to **Restart the Program** from the Floor Menu, sign in again, and go to the Nurses' Station to access the map.) When you click the **Map** icon, a floor map appears, showing the layout of the floor you are currently on, as well as a directory of the patients and services on that floor. As you move your cursor over the directory list, the location of each room is highlighted on the map (and vice versa). The floor map can be accessed from the Nurses' Station, Medication Room, and each patient's room.

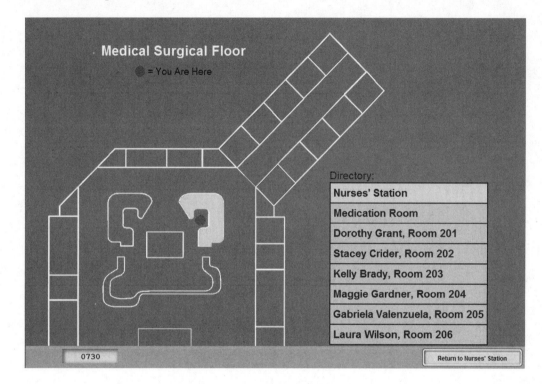

A DETAILED TOUR

If you wish to more thoroughly understand the capabilities of *Virtual Clinical Excursions—Obstetrics-Pediatrics*, take a detailed tour by completing the following section. During this tour, we will work with a specific patient to introduce you to all the different components and learning opportunities available within the software.

■ WORKING WITH A PATIENT

Sign in to work on the Obstetrics Floor for Period of Care 1 (0730-0815). From the Patient List, select Dorothy Grant in Room 201; however, do not go to the Nurses' Station yet.

Patient List

	Patient Name	Room	MRN	Clinical Report
☑	Dorothy Grant	201	1868096	Get Report
☐	Stacey Crider	202	1868065	Get Report
☐	Kelly Brady	203	1868073	Get Report
☐	Maggie Gardner	204	1868085	Get Report
☐	Gabriela Valenzuela	205	1868090	Get Report
☐	Laura Wilson	206	1868098	Get Report

Please select all the patients you will be caring for this period of care. Once you have exited the patient list, you will not be able to change your current selections or select new patients to care for.

0730   Go to Nurses' Station

■ REPORT

In hospitals, when one shift ends and another begins, the outgoing nurse who attended a patient will give a verbal and sometimes a written summary of that patient's condition to the incoming nurse who will assume care for the patient. This summary is called a report and is an important source of data to provide an overview of a patient. Your first task is to get the clinical report on Dorothy Grant. To do this, click **Get Report** in the far right column in this patient's row. From a brief review of this summary, identify the problems and areas of concern that you will need to address for this patient.

When you have finished noting any areas of concern, click **Go to Nurses' Station**.

■ CHARTS

You can access Dorothy Grant's chart from the Nurses' Station or from the patient's room (201). From the Nurses' Station, click on the chart rack or on the **Chart** icon in the tool bar at the top of your screen. Next, click on the chart labeled **201** to open the medical record for Dorothy Grant. Click on the **Emergency Department** tab to view a record of why this patient was admitted.

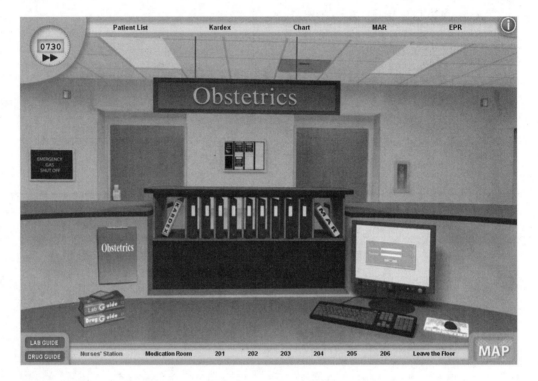

How many days has Dorothy Grant been in the hospital?

What tests were done upon her arrival in the Emergency Department and why?

What was the reason for her admission?

You should also click on **Diagnostic Reports** to learn what additional tests or procedures were performed and when. Finally, review the **Nursing Admission** and **History and Physical** to learn about the health history of this patient. When you are done reviewing the chart, click **Return to Nurses' Station**.

■ **MEDICATIONS**

Open the Medication Administration Record (MAR) by clicking on the **MAR** icon in the tool bar at the top of your screen. *Remember:* The MAR automatically opens to the first occupied room number on the floor—which is not necessarily your patient's room number! Since you need to access Dorothy Grant's MAR, click on tab **201** (her room number). Always make sure you are giving the *Right Drug to the Right Patient!*

Examine the list of medications ordered for Dorothy Grant. In the table below, list the medications that need to be given during this period of care (0730-0815). For each medication, note the dosage, route, and time to be given.

Time	Medication	Dosage	Route

Click on **Return to Nurses' Station**. Next, click on **201** on the bottom tool bar and then verify that you are indeed in Dorothy Grant's room. Select **Clinical Alerts** (the icon to the right of Initial Observations) to check for any emerging data that might affect your medication administration priorities. Next, go to the patient's chart (click on the **Chart** icon; then click on **201**). When the chart opens, select the **Physician's Orders** tab.

Review the orders. Have any new medications been ordered? Return to the MAR (click **Return to Room 201**; then click **MAR**). Verify that any new medications have been correctly transcribed to the MAR. Mistakes are sometimes made in the transcription process in the hospital setting, and it is sound practice to double-check any new order.

Are there any patient assessments you will need to perform before administering these medications? If so, return to Room 201 and click on **Patient Care** and then **Physical Assessment** to complete those assessments before proceeding.

Now click on the **Medication Room** icon in the tool bar at the bottom of your screen to locate and prepare the medications for Dorothy Grant.

In the Medication Room, you must access the medications for Dorothy Grant from the specific dispensing system in which each medication is stored. Locate each medication that needs to be given in this time period and click on **Put Medication on Tray** as appropriate. (*Hint:* Look in **Unit Dosage** drawer first.) When you are finished, click on **Close Drawer** and then on **View Medication Room**. Now click on the medication tray on the counter on the left side of the medication room screen to begin preparing the medications you have selected. (*Remember:* You can also click **Preparation** in the tool bar at the top of screen.)

In the preparation area, you should see a list of the medications you put on the tray in the previous steps. Click on the first medication and then click **Prepare**. Follow the onscreen instructions of the Preparation Wizard, providing any data requested. As an example, let's follow the preparation process for betamethasone, one of the medications due to be administered to Dorothy Grant during this period of care. To begin, click on **Betamethasone**; then click **Prepare**. Now work through the Preparation Wizard sequence as detailed below:

>   Amount of medication in the ampule: 5 mL.
>   Enter the amount of medication you will draw up into a syringe: **3** mL.
>   Click **Next**.
>   Select the patient you wish to set aside the medication for: **Room 201, Dorothy Grant**.
>   Click **Finish**.
>   Click **Return to Medication Room**.

Preparation Wizard

Select the patient you wish to set aside the medication for:

- Room 201, Dorothy Grant
- **Room 202, Stacey Crider**
- **Room 203, Kelly Brady**
- **Room 204, Maggie Gardner**
- Room 205, Gabriela Valenzuela

Confirm that the information contained on the medication label (to the right) is correct and press "Finish" to prepare the medication.

Any leftover medication will be moved to the "leftover" list in your medication lists and can be disposed of or put back into medication systems from there.

Previous   Finish

Medication set aside for:
Room 201, Dorothy Grant

Betamethasone
Strength: 4 mg/mL
Units: 1 syringe
Dosage/Unit: 3 mL/syringe

CLOSE

LAB GUIDE   DRUG GUIDE   0734   Review MAR   Review Your Medications   View Medication Room

Follow this same basic process for the other medications due to be administered to Dorothy Grant during this period of care. (*Hint:* Look in **IV Storage** and **Automated System**.)

PREPARATION WIZARD EXCEPTIONS

- Some medications in *Virtual Clinical Excursions—Obstetrics-Pediatrics* are prepared by the pharmacy (e.g., IV antibiotics) and taken to the patient room as a whole. This is common practice in most hospitals.
- Blood products are not administered by students through the *Virtual Clinical Excursions—Obstetrics-Pediatrics* simulations since blood administration follows specific protocols not covered in this program.
- The *Virtual Clinical Excursions—Obstetrics-Pediatrics* simulations do not allow for mixing more than one type of medication, such as regular and Lente insulins, in the same syringe. In the clinical setting, when multiple types of insulin are ordered for a patient, the regular insulin is drawn up first, followed by the longer-acting insulin. Insulin is always administered in a special unit-marked syringe.

Now return to Room 201 (click on **201** on the bottom tool bar) to administer Dorothy Grant's medications.

At any time during the medication administration process, you can perform a further review of systems, take vital signs, check information contained within the chart, or verify patient identity and allergies. Inside Dorothy Grant's room, click **Take Vital Signs**. (*Note:* These findings change over time to reflect the temporal changes you would find in a patient similar to Dorothy Grant.)

When you have gathered all the data you need, click on **Patient Care** and then select **Medication Administration**. Any medications you prepared in the previous steps should be listed on the left side of your screen. Let's continue the administration process with the betamethasone ordered for Dorothy Grant. Click to highlight **Betamethasone** in the list of medications. Next, click on the down arrow to the right of **Select** and choose **Administer** from the drop-down menu. This will activate the Administration Wizard. Complete the Wizard sequence as follows:

- Route: **Injection**
- Method: **Intramuscular**
- Site: **Any**
- Click **Administer to Patient** arrow.
- Would you like to document this administration in the MAR? **Yes**
- Click **Finish** arrow.

Your selections are recorded by a tracking system and evaluated on a Medication Scorecard stored under Preceptor's Evaluations. This scorecard can be viewed, printed, and given to your instructor. To access the Preceptor's Evaluations, click on **Leave the Floor**. When the Floor Menu appears, select **Look at Your Preceptor's Evaluation**. Then click on **Medication Scorecard** inside the box with Dorothy Grant's name (see example on the following page).

MEDICATION SCORECARD

- First, review Table A. Was betamethasone given correctly? Did you give the other medications as ordered?
- Table B shows you which (if any) medications you gave incorrectly.
- Table C addresses the resources used for Dorothy Grant. Did you access the patient's chart, MAR, EPR, or Kardex as needed to make safe medication administration decisions?
- Did you check the patient's armband to verify her identity? Did you check whether your patient had any known allergies to medications? Were vital signs taken?

When you have finished reviewing the scorecard, click **Return to Evaluations** and then **Return to Menu**.

■ VITAL SIGNS

Vital signs, often considered the traditional "signs of life," include body temperature, heart rate, respiratory rate, blood pressure, oxygen saturation of the blood, and pain level.

Inside Dorothy Grant's room, click **Take Vital Signs**. (*Note:* If you are following this detailed tour step by step, you will need to **Restart the Program** from the Floor Menu, sign in again for Period of Care 1, and navigate to Room 201.) Collect vital signs for this patient and record them below. Note the time at which you collected each of these data. (*Remember:* You can take vital signs at any time. The data change over time to reflect the temporal changes you would find in a patient similar to Dorothy Grant.)

Vital Signs	Findings/Time
Blood pressure	
O$_2$ saturation	
Temperature	
Heart rate	
Respiratory rate	
Pain rating	

After you are done, click on the **EPR** icon located in the tool bar at the top of the screen. Your username and password are automatically provided. Click on **Login** to enter the EPR. To access Dorothy Grant's records, click on the down arrow next to Patient and choose her room number, **201**. Select **Vital Signs** as the category. Next, in the empty time column on the far right, record the vital signs data you just collected in the patient's room. If you need help with this process, refer to the Electronic Patient Record (EPR) section of the Quick Tour. Now compare these findings with the data you collected earlier for this patient's vital signs. Use these earlier findings to establish a baseline for each of the vital signs.

    a.   Are any of the data you collected significantly different from the baseline for a particular vital sign?

        Circle One: Yes   No

    b.   If "Yes," which data are different?

■ PHYSICAL ASSESSMENT

After you have finished examining the EPR for vital signs, click **Exit EPR** to return to Room 201. Click **Patient Care** and then **Physical Assessment**. Think about the information you received in the report at the beginning of this shift, as well as what you may have learned about this patient from the chart. Based on this, what area(s) of examination should you pay most attention to at this time? Is there any equipment you should be monitoring? Conduct a physical assessment of the body areas and systems that you consider priorities for Dorothy Grant. For example, select **Head & Neck**; then click on and assess **Sensory** and **Lymphatic**. Complete any other assessment(s) you think are necessary at this time. In the following table, record the data you collected during this examination.

Area of Examination	Findings
Head & Neck Sensory	
Head & Neck Lymphatic	

After you have finished collecting these data, return to the EPR. Compare the data that were already in the record with those you just collected.

a. Are any of the data you collected significantly different from the baselines for this patient?

Circle One: Yes   No

b. If "Yes," which data are different?

■ NURSE-CLIENT INTERACTIONS

Click on **Patient Care** from inside Dorothy Grant's room (201). Now click on **Nurse-Client Interactions** to access a short video titled **Patient Teaching—Medication**, which is available for viewing at or after 0730 (based on the virtual clock in the upper left corner of your screen; see *Note* below). To begin the video, click on the white arrow next to its title. You will observe a nurse communicating with Dorothy Grant. There are many variations of nursing practice, some exemplifying "best" practice and some not. Note whether the nurse in this interaction displays professional behavior and compassionate care. Are her words congruent with what is going on with the patient? Does this interaction "feel right" to you? If not, how would you handle this situation differently? Explain.

Note: If the video you wish to view is not listed, this means you have not yet reached the correct virtual time to view that video. Check the virtual clock; you may return to access the video once its designated time has occurred—as long as you do so within the same period of care. Or you can click on the fast-forward icon within the virtual clock to advance the time by 2-minute intervals. You will then need to click again on **Patient Care** and **Nurse-Client Interactions** to refresh the screen.

At least one Nurse-Client Interactions video is available during each period of care. Viewing these videos can help you learn more about what is occurring with a patient at a certain time and also prompt you to discern between nurse communications that are ideal and those that need improvement. Compassionate care and the ability to communicate clearly are essential components of delivering quality nursing care, and it is during your clinical time that you will begin to refine these skills.

■ COLLECTING AND EVALUATING DATA

Each of the activities you perform in the Patient Care environment generates a significant amount of assessment data. Remember that after you collect data, you can record your findings in the EPR. You can also review the EPR, patient's chart, videos, and MAR at any time. You will get plenty of practice collecting and then evaluating data in context of the patient's course.

Now, here's an important question for you:

> Did the previous sequence of exercises provide the most efficient way to assess Dorothy Grant?

For example, you went to the patient's room to get vital signs, then back to the EPR to enter data and compare your findings with extant data. Next, you went back to the patient's room to do a physical examination, then again back to the EPR to enter and review data. If this back-and-forth process of data collection and recording seemed inefficient, remember the following:

- Plan all of your nursing activities to maximize efficiency, while at the same time optimizing the quality of patient care. (Think about what data you might need before performing certain tasks. For example, do you need to check a heart rate before administering a cardiac medication or check an IV site before starting an infusion?)

- You collect a tremendous amount of data when you work with a patient. Very few people can accurately remember all these data for more than a few minutes. Develop efficient assessment skills, and record data as soon as possible after collecting them.

- Assessment data are only the starting point for the nursing process.

Make a clear distinction between these first exercises and how you actually provide nursing care. These initial exercises were designed to involve you actively in the use of different software components. This workbook focuses on sensible practices for implementing the nursing process in ways that ensure the highest-quality care of patients.

Most important, remember that a human being changes through time, and that these changes include both the physical and psychosocial facets of a person as a living organism. Think about this for a moment. Some patients may change physically in a very short time (a patient with emerging myocardial infarction) or more slowly (a patient with a chronic illness). Patients' overall physical and psychosocial conditions may improve or deteriorate. They may have effective coping skills and familial support, or they may feel alone and full of despair. In fact, each individual is a complex mix of physical and psychosocial elements, and at least some of these elements usually change through time.

Thus it is crucial that you *DO NOT* think of the nursing process as a simple one-time, five-step procedure consisting of assessment, nursing diagnosis, planning, implementation, and evaluation. Rather, the nursing process should be utilized as a creative and systematic approach to delivering nursing care. Furthermore, because all living organisms are constantly changing, we must apply the nursing process over and over. Each time we follow the nursing process for an individual patient, we refine our understanding of that patient's physical and psychosocial conditions based on collection and analysis of many different types of data. *Virtual Clinical Excursions—Obstetrics-Pediatrics* will help you develop both the creativity and the systematic approach needed to become a nurse who is equipped to deliver the highest-quality care to all patients.

REDUCING MEDICATION ERRORS

Earlier in the detailed tour, you learned the basic steps of medication preparation and administration. The following simulations will allow you to practice those skills further—with an increased emphasis on reducing medication errors by using the Medication Scorecard to evaluate your work.

Sign in to work on the Obstetrics Floor at Pacific View Regional Hospital for Period of Care 1. (*Note:* If you are already working with another patient or during another period of care, click on **Leave the Floor** and then **Restart the Program**; then sign in.)

From the Patient List, select Dorothy Grant. Then click on **Go to Nurses' Station**. Complete the following steps to prepare and administer medications to Dorothy Grant.

- Click on **Medication Room** on the tool bar at the bottom of your screen.
- Click on **MAR** and then on tab **201** to determine medications that have been ordered for Dorothy Grant. (*Note:* You may click on **Review MAR** at any time to verify the correct medication order. Always remember to check the patient name on the MAR to make sure you have the correct patient's record. You must click on the correct room number tab within the MAR.) Click on **Return to Medication Room** after reviewing the correct MAR.
- Click on **Unit Dosage** (or on the Unit Dosage cabinet); from the close-up view, click on drawer **201**.
- Select the medications you would like to administer. After each selection, click **Put Medication on Tray**. When you are finished selecting medications, click **Close Drawer** and then **View Medication Room**.
- Click **Automated System** (or on the Automated System unit itself). Click **Login**.
- On the next screen, specify the correct patient and drawer location.
- Select the medication you would like to administer and click **Put Medication on Tray**. Repeat this process if you wish to administer other medications from the Automated System.
- When you are finished, click **Close Drawer** and **View Medication Room**.
- From the Medication Room, click **Preparation** (or on the preparation tray).
- From the list of medications on your tray, highlight the correct medication to administer and click **Prepare**.
- This activates the Preparation Wizard. Supply any requested information; then click **Next**.
- Now select the correct patient to receive this medication and click **Finish**.
- Repeat the previous three steps until all medications that you want to administer are prepared.
- You can click on **Review Your Medications** and then on **Return to Medication Room** when ready. Once you are back in the Medication Room, go directly to Dorothy Grant's room by clicking on **201** at the bottom of the screen.
- Inside the patient's room, administer the medication, utilizing the six rights of medication administration. After you have collected the appropriate assessment data and are ready for administration, click **Patient Care** and then **Medication Administration**. Verify that the correct patient and medication(s) appear in the left-hand window. Highlight the first medication you wish to administer; then click the down arrow next to Select. From the drop-down menu, select **Administer** and complete the Administration Wizard by providing any information requested. When the Wizard stops asking for information, click **Administer to Patient**. Specify **Yes** when asked whether this administration should be recorded in the MAR. Finally, click **Finish**.

■ SELF-EVALUATION

Now let's see how you did during your medication administration!

- Click on **Leave the Floor** at the bottom of your screen. From the Floor Menu, select **Look at Your Preceptor's Evaluation**. Then click **Medication Scorecard**.

The following exercises will help you identify medication errors, investigate possible reasons for these errors, and reduce or prevent medication errors in the future.

1. Start by examining Table A. These are the medications you should have given to Dorothy Grant during this period of care. If each of the medications in Table A has a ✓ by it, then you made no errors. Congratulations!

If any medication has an X by it, then you made one or more medication errors.

Compare Tables A and B to determine which of the following types of errors you made: Wrong Dose, Wrong Route/Method/Site, or Wrong Time. Follow these steps:
   a. Find medications in Table A that were given incorrectly.
   b. Now see if those same medications are in Table B, which shows what you actually administered to Dorothy Grant.
   c. Comparing Tables A and B, match the Strength, Dose, Route/Method/Site, and Time for each medication you administered incorrectly.
   d. Then, using the form below, list the medications given incorrectly and mark the errors you made for each medication.

Medication	Strength	Dosage	Route	Method	Site	Time
	❑	❑	❑	❑	❑	❑
	❑	❑	❑	❑	❑	❑
	❑	❑	❑	❑	❑	❑
	❑	❑	❑	❑	❑	❑

2. To help you reduce future medication errors, consider the following list of possible reasons for errors.

- Did not check drug against MAR for correct medication, correct dose, correct patient, correct route, correct time, correct documentation.
- Did not check drug dose against MAR three times.
- Did not open the unit dose package in the patient's room.
- Did not correctly identify the patient using two identifiers.
- Did not administer the drug on time.
- Did not verify patient allergies.
- Did not check the patient's current condition or vital sign parameters.
- Did not consider why the patient would be receiving this drug.
- Did not question why the drug was in the patient's drawer.
- Did not check the physician's order and/or check with the pharmacist when there was a question about the drug or dose.
- Did not verify that no adverse effects had occurred from a previous dose.

Based on the list of possibilities you just reviewed, determine how you made each error and record the reason in the form below:

Medication	Reason for Error

3. Look again at Table B. Are there medications listed that are not in Table A? If so, you gave a medication to Dorothy Grant that she should not have received. Complete the following exercises to help you understand how such an error might have been made.

   a. Perhaps you gave a medication that was on Dorothy Grant's MAR for this period of care, without recognizing that a change had occurred in the patient's condition, which should have caused you to reconsider. Review patient records as necessary and complete the following form:

Medication	Possible Reasons Not to Give This Medication

   b. Another possibility is that you gave Dorothy Grant a medication that should have been given at a different time. Check her MAR and complete the form below to determine whether you made a Wrong Time error:

Medication	Given to Dorothy Grant at What Time	Should Have Been Given at What Time

c. Maybe you gave another patient's medication to Dorothy Grant. In this case, you made a Wrong Patient error. Check the MARs of other patients and use the form below to determine whether you made this type of error:

Medication	Given to Dorothy Grant	Should Have Been Given to

4. The Medication Scorecard provides some other interesting sources of information. For example, if there is a medication selected for Dorothy Grant but it was not given to her, there will be an X by that medication in Table A, but it will not appear in Table B. In that case, you might have given this medication to some other patient, which is another type of Wrong Patient error. To investigate further, look at Table D, which lists the medications you gave to other patients. See whether you can find any medications ordered for Dorothy Grant that were given to another patient by mistake. However, before you make any decisions, be sure to cross-check the MAR for other patients because the same medication may have been ordered for multiple patients. Use the following form to record your findings:

Medication	Should Have Been Given to Dorothy Grant	Given by Mistake to

5. Now take some time to review the medication exercises you just completed. Use the form below to create an overall analysis of what you have learned. Once again, record each of the medication errors you made, including the type of each error. Then, for each error you made, indicate specifically what you would do differently to prevent this type of error from occurring again.

Medication	Type of Error	Error Prevention Tactic

Submit this form to your instructor if required as a graded assignment, or simply use these exercises to improve your understanding of medication errors and how to reduce them.

Name: _____   Date: _____

Prenatal Assessment, Care, and Nutrition

Reading Assignment: Prenatal Care and Adaptations to Pregnancy (Chapter 4)
Nursing Care of Women with Complications During Pregnancy (Chapter 5)

Patients: Kelly Brady, Obstetrics Floor, Room 203
Maggie Gardner, Obstetrics Floor, Room 204

Objectives:

1. Differentiate between the various types of assessment techniques that can be used with low- and high-risk pregnancy patients.
2. Identify appropriate interventions for maintaining adequate maternal and fetal nutrition.
3. Discuss the physiological changes of pregnancy.
4. Identify various methods of testing that can be used in high-risk pregnancies.

Exercise 1

Virtual Hospital Activity

30 minutes

1. Match the prenatal tests below with the trimester in which they are normally performed.

Prenatal Test	**Trimester**
_____ Blood type and RH antibody screen	a. First trimester
_____ Serum alpha fetoprotein	b. Second trimester
_____ Amniocentesis	c. Third trimester
_____ Cervical fibronectin assay	
_____ Blood glucose screen	
_____ Rubella titer	
_____ VDRL	
_____ Real-time ultrasonography	
_____ Group B streptococcus	

2. The nurse is preparing to calculate an assigned patient's estimated date of delivery. What will the nurse need to do? Select all that apply.

   _____ Determine the number of days the last menstrual period lasted.

   _____ Determine the first day of the last menstrual period.

   _____ Count backward 3 months from the first day of the last menstrual period.

   _____ Add 10 days to the first day of the last menstrual period.

   _____ Determine the last day of the last menstrual period.

3. Match each pregnancy-related hormone below with its correct description.

Hormone	Description
_____ Estrogen	a. Stimulates uterine contractions
_____ Progesterone	b. Prepares the breasts for lactation
_____ Relaxin	c. Encourages enlargement of the uterus
_____ Human placental lactogen	d. Stimulates estrogen and progesterone production early in the pregnancy to sustain the pregnancy until the placenta begins to function
_____ Human chorionic gonadotropin	
_____ Oxytocin	e. Remodels collagen, causing connective tissue of symphysis pubis to be more
_____ Prolactin	f. Reduces smooth muscle tone
	g. Impacts glucose and protein metabolism

4. List the danger signs that pregnant women must be advised to report.

5. The nurse is reviewing the symptoms of a women suspected of being pregnant. Which symptoms and/or signs can be characterized as probable? Select all that apply.

_____ Heger's sign

_____ Amenorrhea

_____ Nausea and vomiting

_____ Positive serum pregnancy test

_____ Positive urine pregnancy test

_____ Urinary frequency

_____ Goodell's sign

- Sign in to work at Pacific View Regional Hospital on the Obstetrics Floor for Period of Care 3. (*Note:* If you are already in the virtual hospital from a previous exercise, click on **Leave the Floor** and then on **Restart the Program** to get to the sign-in window.)
- From the Patient List, select Maggie Gardner (Room 204).
- Click on **Go to Nurses' Station**.
- Click on **Chart** and then on **204** to view Maggie Gardner's chart.
- Click on the **History and Physical** tab and review the information given.
- Click on the **Diagnostic Reports** tab and review the information given.

6. Which terms correctly apply to Maggie Gardner's obstetrical history? Select all that apply.

_____ Primigravida

_____ Primipara

_____ Nullipara

_____ Multigravida

7. Complete the following obstetrical history for Maggie Gardner using the acronym TPALM.

T =

P =

A =

L =

M =

8. According to the Diagnostic Report, Maggie Gardner had an _____ ultrasound

with _____.

9. Based on the ultrasound findings, how large is the baby?

10. List three abnormalities found on Maggie Gardner's ultrasound in regard to the placenta.

11. What is the impression from Maggie Gardner's ultrasound in terms of the fetus and the placenta?

12. What are the recommendations regarding follow-up?

13. When estimating the fetal age of Maggie Gardner's baby, what measurements will likely be used? Select all that apply.

_____ Biparietal diameter

_____ Crown rump length

_____ Femur length

_____ Abdominal circumference

_____ Radial bone diameter

Exercise 2

Virtual Hospital Activity

30 minutes

Read about biophysical profiles in your textbook.

1. A biophysical profile is one of several tools used to assess fetal well-being during a high-risk pregnancy. What items are assessed with this test? Select all that apply.

   _____ Fetal breathing movements

   _____ Fetal size

   _____ Fetal body movements

   _____ Fetal tone

   _____ Fetal gestational age

   _____ Fetal heart rate and reactivity (NST)

   _____ Amniotic fluid volume

   _____ Fetal lung maturity

2. What tests are incorporated into the biophysical profile? Select all that apply.

   _____ Nonstress test

   _____ Stress test

   _____ Amniocentesis

   _____ Ultrasound

   _____ Chorionic villus sampling

3. A biophysical profile is used to identify reduced fetal _____ in

   conditions associated with poor _____ function.

4. _____ In the presence of fetal hypoxia, fetal tone is lost first. (True/False)

5. Amniotic fluid volume is _____ when placental function is poor.

- Sign in to work at Pacific View Regional Hospital on the Obstetrics Floor for Period of Care 3. (*Note:* If you are already in the virtual hospital from a previous exercise, click on **Leave the Floor** and then on **Restart the Program** to get to the sign-in window.)
- From the Patient List, select Kelly Brady (Room 203).
- Click on **Go to Nurses' Station**.
- Click on **Chart** and then on **203** to view Kelly Brady's chart.
- Click on the **History and Physical** tab and review the information given.
- Click on the **Diagnostic Reports** tab and review the information given.

6. What is the estimated gestational age of Kelly Brady's fetus?

7. Using Kelly Brady's last menstrual period (LMP) calculate her EDD.
   a. January 22
   b. February 1
   c. January 15
   d. February 14

8. What is the amniotic fluid index as indicated in the Diagnostic Report?

9. If there were an abnormal amniotic fluid index indicated on Kelly Brady's report, what might that indicate?

10. What is the normal size of a pocket of amniotic fluid?

11. What measurement would indicate oligohydramnios? Polyhydramnios?

Exercise 3

Virtual Hospital Activity

30 minutes

- Sign in to work at Pacific View Regional Hospital on the Obstetrics Floor for Period of Care 1. (*Note:* If you are already in the virtual hospital from a previous exercise, click on **Leave the Floor** and then on **Restart the Program** to get to the sign-in window.)
- From the Patient List, select Maggie Gardner (Room 204).
- Click on **Go to Nurses' Station**.
- Click on **Chart** and then on **204** to view Maggie Gardner's chart.
- Click on the **Laboratory Reports** tab and review the information given.

Review information regarding anemia in your textbook.

1. What are Maggie Gardner's hemoglobin and hematocrit levels?

- Click on the **History and Physical** tab in Maggie Gardner's chart.

2. What puts Maggie Gardner at a greater risk for developing anemia than the average pregnancy patient? (*Hint:* Review the Genetic Screening section of her History and Physical.)

3. What is the recommended daily intake of iron for pregnant women?
   a. 15 mg
   b. 25 mg
   c. 30 mg
   d. 35 mg

4. What is a normal hemoglobin level for a woman who is pregnant?

5. What assessments specifically related to an anemia diagnosis need to be performed by the nurse at each visit?

6. What are some sources of iron that you could encourage Maggie Gardner to add to her diet?

7. When providing dietary education to Maggie Smith, what information about iron intake should be included? Select all that apply.

_____ Taking iron with food will promote its absorption.

_____ Citrus beverages improve iron absorption by the body.

_____ Taking iron on an empty stomach will help limit possible GI upset.

_____ Avoid taking iron supplements with milk.

_____ Avoid taking iron supplements with caffeine-containing beverages.

8. When reviewing Maggie Gardner's diet, what daily quantity of meat and beans is recommended?
   a. 4 ounces
   b. 6.5 ounces
   d. 7.5 ounces
   d. 8 ounces

9. Maggie Gardner's weight is 180 pounds. She is 5 feet 6 inches tall. Her BMI before pregnancy was greater than 26. How much weight is she recommended to gain?
   a. 11-15 pounds
   b. 11-25 pounds
   c. 25-35 pounds
   d. 28-40 pounds

10. How much weight has Maggie Gardner gained so far with this pregnancy?

LESSON 2

Nursing Care of Women with Complications During Pregnancy: Antepartal Bleeding Disorders

Reading Assignment: Prenatal Care and Adaptations to Pregnancy (Chapter 4)
Nursing Care of Women with Complications During Pregnancy (Chapter 5)
Nursing Care of Women with Complications During Labor and Birth
 (Chapter 8)
Health Care Adaptations for the Child and Family (Chapter 22)

Patient: Gabriela Valenzuela, Obstetrics Floor, Room 205

Objectives:

1. Differentiate between the symptoms of abruptio placentae and those of placenta previa.
2. Identify appropriate interventions for managing abruptio placentae.
3. Plan and evaluate essential patient education during the acute phase of diagnosis.

Exercise 1

Virtual Hospital Activity

15 minutes

- Sign in to work at Pacific View Regional Hospital on the Obstetrics Floor for Period of Care 1. (*Note:* If you are already in the virtual hospital from a previous exercise, click on **Leave the Floor** and then on **Restart the Program** to get to the sign-in window.)
- From the Patient List, select Gabriela Valenzuela (Room 205).
- Click on **Go to Nurses' Station**.
- Click on **Chart** and then on **205**.
- Click on the **Emergency Department** tab and review the information given.

1. What brought Gabriela Valenzuela to the Emergency Department? How long did she wait to come, and what was the deciding factor in her coming to the Emergency Department?

Read about the incidence and etiology of abruptio placentae in your textbook.

2. Which are considered risk factors for the development of abruptio placentae? Select all that apply.

_____ Maternal hypotension

_____ Cocaine use

_____ Abdominal trauma

_____ Obesity

_____ Iron deficiency

_____ Poor nutrition

3. Differential diagnosis is very important when a patient presents with clinical manifestations that could be evidence of more than one process. Complete the following table by comparing abruptio placentae and placenta previa. (*Hint:* See Table 5-4 in your textbook.)

Characteristic/ Complication	Placenta Previa	Abruptio Placentae
Bleeding		
Blood clotting		
Uterine tonicity		
Tenderness/pain		

Characteristic/ Complication	Placenta Previa	Abruptio Placentae
Placenta findings		
Fetal		

4. Review Gabriela Valenzuela's Emergency Department records. What type of abruption is Gabriela Valenzuela most likely to have, given the information in this record?
   a. Partial
   b. Marginal
   c. Total
   d. Incomplete

- Click on **Return to Nurses' Station** and then on **205** at the bottom of the screen to go to the patient's room.
- Inside the room, click on **Patient Care** and then on **Nurse-Client Interactions**.
- Select and view the video titled **0740: Patient Teaching—Fetal Monitor**. (*Note:* Check the virtual clock to see whether enough time has elapsed. You can use the fast-forward feature to advance the time by 2-minute intervals if the video is not yet available. Then click again on **Patient Care** and **Nurse-Client Interactions** to refresh the screen.)

5. Once Gabriela Valenzuela is admitted to the floor, what are her and her husband's concerns? What does the nurse include in her teaching to alleviate those concerns?

- Select and view the video titled **0805: Patient Teaching—Abruption**. (*Note:* Check the virtual clock to see whether enough time has elapsed. You can use the fast-forward feature to advance the time by 2-minute intervals if the video is not yet available. Then click again on **Patient Care** and **Nurse-Client Interactions** to refresh the screen.)

6. What interventions will help to increase the oxygen supply to the baby and prevent further separation of the placenta?
   a. Placing the patient on her left side
   b. Placing the patient in a prone position
   c. Placing the patient in Trendelenburg position
   d. Placing the patient in a lithotomy position

Exercise 2

Virtual Hospital Activity

20 minutes

- Sign in to work at Pacific View Regional Hospital on the Obstetrics Floor for Period of Care 1. (*Note:* If you are already in the virtual hospital from a previous exercise, click on **Leave the Floor** and then on **Restart the Program** to get to the sign-in window.)
- From the Patient List, select Gabriela Valenzuela (Room 205).
- Click on **Go to Nurses' Station**.

Gabriela Valenzuela is at increased risk for early delivery as a result of her earlier abdominal trauma and the subsequent occurrence of a grade 1 abruptio placentae. She is currently manifesting signs and symptoms of early labor. According to the Emergency Department notes, she was given a dose of betamethasone, which was to be repeated in 12 hours.

1. Betamethasone has been prescribed for Gabriela Valenzuela. What is the purpose of the administration of this medication in this situation?

- Click on the **Drug** icon in the lower left-hand corner of your screen.
- Use the search box to locate information for betamethasone.

2. Based on the information provided in the Drug Guide, what is the indication and dosage of betamethasone for pregnant adults?

- Click on **Return to Nurses' Station**
- Click on **MAR** and then on tab **205**.
- Review the dosage of betamethasone to be given.
- Click on **Return to Nurses' Station** and then on **Medication Room** at the bottom of the screen.
- Click on **Unit Dosage** and then on drawer **205**.
- Click on **Betamethasone**; then click on **Put Medication on Tray**.
- Click on **Close Drawer**.
- Click on **View Medication Room** and then on **Preparation**.

- Click on **Prepare** next to betamethasone and follow the prompts of the Preparation Wizard.
- Click on **Return to Medication Room** and then on **205** at the bottom of the screen to go to the patient's room.
- Inside the room, click on **Patient Care** and then on **Medication Administration**.
- Click on **Review Your Medications** and then click on the **Prepared** tab.

3. According to the box on the right side of your screen, what is the medication name and dosage that you have prepared for Gabriela Valenzuela?

4. Based on your answer to question 2, how many mg are you giving to Gabriela Valenzuela? Is this the correct dosage based on the MAR?

- Click on **Return to Room 205**.
- Click on the **Drug** icon in the lower left-hand corner of your screen.
- Use the search box or scroll down the list of medications to find betamethasone.

5. After reviewing the information in the Drug Guide regarding betamethasone, which assessments need to be included in the plan of care for Gabriela Valenzuela? Select all that apply.

_____ Assess baseline temperature

_____ Assess baseline blood pressure

_____ Review for history of diabetes

_____ Monitor complete blood count results for alterations in white blood cell count

_____ Review medication history for potential drug interactions with betamethasone

6. Review the information regarding the administration of betamethasone. What are three things that must be taken into consideration when giving this medication in the injection form?

7. After the administration of betamethasone, what potential side effects may Gabriela Valenzuela experience? Select all that apply.

_____ Anorexia

_____ Nervousness

_____ Sleepiness

_____ Pruritus

_____ Stinging at injection site

8. What are the six rights of medication administration?

(1)

(2)

(3)

(4)

(5)

(6)

Now you are ready to complete the medication administration.

- Click on **Return to Room 205**.
- Click on **Check Armband**.
- Click on **Patient Care** and then on **Medication Administration**.
- View the medications set aside for Gabriela Valenzuela.
- Click on the drop-down box next to betamethasone, select **Administer**, and follow the prompts to administer Gabriela Valenzuela's betamethasone.
- Document the injection in the MAR.
- Click on **Leave the Floor** and then on **Look at Your Preceptor's Evaluation**.
- Click on **Medication Scorecard**. How did you do?
- Click on **Return to Evaluations** and then on **Return to Menu**.

Exercise 3

Virtual Hospital Activity

20 minutes

- Sign in to work at Pacific View Regional Hospital on the Obstetrics Floor for Period of Care 2. (*Note:* If you are already in the virtual hospital from a previous exercise, click on **Leave the Floor** and then on **Restart the Program** to get to the sign-in window.)
- From the Patient List, select Gabriela Valenzuela (Room 205).
- Click on **Go to Nurses' Station**.

- Click on **Chart** and then on **205**.
- Click on the **Diagnostic Reports** tab and review the information given.

1. Gabriela Valenzuela had an ultrasound on Tuesday to determine the source of her bleeding. What were the findings of the ultrasound?

- Click on the **Laboratory Reports** tab and review the results.

2. What are Gabriela Valenzuela's hemoglobin and hematocrit levels on Tuesday? How does this compare with Wednesday's report? Is there a significant change?

3. According to the textbook, the hematocrit level of a pregnant patient should be between

_____% and _____%.

4. What clinical manifestations would indicate that there is a worsening in the condition of either the patient or the fetus?

- Click on **Return to Nurses' Station**.
- Click on **EPR** and then on **Login**.
- Select **205** for the Patient and then select **Vital Signs** from the Category drop-down menu.
- Using the right and left arrows, scroll to review Gabriela Valenzuela's vital signs over the last 12 hours.

5. Based on her vital signs from 0000 Wednesday to 1200 Wednesday, would you consider Gabriela Valenzuela's condition stable or unstable? What is your rationale?

- Click on **Exit EPR**.
- Click on **205** at the bottom of the screen.
- Click on **Patient Care** and then on **Nurse-Client Interactions**.
- Select and view the video titled **1140: Intervention—Bleeding, Comfort**. Take notes regarding the interaction. (*Note:* Check the virtual clock to see whether enough time has elapsed. You can use the fast-forward feature to advance the time by 2-minute intervals if the video is not yet available. Then click again on **Patient Care** and **Nurse-Client Interactions** to refresh the screen.)

6. What happened that elicited this interaction? (*Hint:* In the patient's chart, review the Nurse's Notes for Wednesday 1140.)

7. What actions did the nurse take during the interaction with the patient? (Include what is documented in the Nurse's Notes.)

Exercise 4

Virtual Hospital Activity

20 minutes

- Sign in to work at Pacific View Regional Hospital on the Obstetrics Floor for Period of Care 3. (*Note:* If you are already in the virtual hospital from a previous exercise, click on **Leave the Floor** and then on **Restart the Program** to get to the sign-in window.)
- From the Patient List, select Gabriela Valenzuela (Room 205).
- Click on **Go to Nurses' Station**.
- Click on **Kardex** and then on tab **205**.

1. What problem areas related to Gabriela Valenzuela's diagnosis have been identified by the nurse?

2. Which problem area is of the highest priority for Gabriela Valenzuela?

3. What is the focus of the expected outcomes related to these problems?

4. Using standard NANDA nursing diagnosis wording and format, write four possible nursing diagnoses for Gabriela Valenzuela.

- Click on **Return to Nurses' Station**.
- Click on **Chart** and then on **205**.
- Click on the **Patient Education** tab and review the information given.

5. According to the patient education sheet in Gabriela Valenzuela's chart, what are the educational goals related to her diagnosis?

- Click on the **Nurse's Notes** tab and review the notes.

6. What patient education has been completed by the nurses from Gabriela Valenzuela's admission through Period of Care 3? Include documentation of times and topics.

7. What are some barriers to learning that the nurse may confront with Gabriela Valenzuela? (*Hint:* Review the Nurse's Notes in the chart.)

8. How can the nurse overcome each of these barriers?

Nursing Care of Women with Complications During Pregnancy: Gestational Hypertension

Reading Assignment: Nursing Care of Women with Complications During Pregnancy (Chapter 5)

Patient: Kelly Brady, Obstetrics Floor, Room 203

Objectives:

1. Compare and contrast the hypertensive conditions of pregnancy.
2. Assess and identify signs and symptoms present in the patient with severe preeclampsia.
3. Explain how the common signs and symptoms present in the patient with severe preeclampsia relate to the underlying pathophysiology of this disease.
4. Identify the patient who has developed HELLP syndrome.
5. Describe routine nursing care for the patient with severe preeclampsia who is receiving magnesium sulfate.

In this lesson you will assess and plan care for a patient with severe preeclampsia who then develops HELLP syndrome and delivers at 26²/₇ weeks gestation.

Exercise 1

Virtual Hospital Activity

15 minutes

- Sign in to work at Pacific View Regional Hospital on the Obstetrics Floor for Period of Care 3. (*Note:* If you are already in the virtual hospital from a previous exercise, click on **Leave the Floor** and then on **Restart the Program** to get to the sign-in window.)
- From the Patient List, select Kelly Brady (Room 203).
- Click on **Go to Nurses' Station**.
- Click on **Chart** and then on **203**.
- Click on the **History and Physical** tab and review the information given.

1. What was Kelly Brady's diagnosis on admission?

2. Identify risk factors from Kelly Brady's medical and obstetrical history that place her at risk for the development of preeclampsia. (*Hint:* Refer to Box 5-3 in your textbook.)

3. Using the History and Physical information from chapter 5 in your textbook, complete the table below.

Sign/ Symptom	Gestational Hypertension	Severe Preeclampsia	Kelly Brady on Admission
Blood pressure			
Proteinuria			
Headache			
Reflexes			
Visual problems			
Epigastric pain			
Edema			

4. Kelly Brady's admission information indicates the signs and symptoms she experienced that are consistent with blood pressure elevations before seeking care. What is traditionally the first symptom noticed by the pregnant patient experiencing hypertension?

• Click on the **Physician's Orders** tab and find the admitting physician's orders on Tuesday at 1030.

5. What tests/procedures did Kelly Brady's physician order to confirm the diagnosis of severe preeclampsia?

6. As a result of her elevated blood pressure, Kelly Brady is at increased risk for developing what complications? Select all that apply.

_____ Placenta previa

_____ Placental abruption

_____ Fetal growth restriction

_____ Prematurity

_____ Stillbirth

_____ Polyhydramnios

7. What diet has the physician prescribed for Kelly Brady? What is the rationale for not restricting sodium?

• Click on the **Physician's Notes** tab and review the note for Wednesday 0730.
• Kelly Brady's 24-hour urine collection was completed and sent to the lab at 1230.
• Click on the **Laboratory Reports** tab and scroll down to review the results for Wednesday 1230.

8. What were the results of Kelly Brady's 24-hour urine collection?

9. When explaining why protein is in the urine of a patient with hypertension in pregnancy, what information should be provided?

Exercise 2

Virtual Hospital Activity

30 minutes

- Sign in to work at Pacific View Regional Hospital on the Obstetrics Floor for Period of Care 1. (*Note:* If you are already in the virtual hospital from a previous exercise, click on **Leave the Floor** and then on **Restart the Program** to get to the sign-in window.)
- From the Patient List, select Kelly Brady (Room 203).
- Click on **Go to Nurses' Station** and then on **203** at the bottom of the screen.
- Click on **Take Vital Signs**.

1. Record Kelly Brady's current vital signs below. (*Note:* Answers will vary depending on the exact time you take them.)

    Temperature:

    Heart rate:

    Respirations:

    Blood pressure:

    Pain rating:

- Click on **Patient Care** and perform a physical assessment by selecting the various body systems (yellow buttons) and body system subcategories (green buttons) as specified in the table in question 2.

2. Record your findings from the focused assessment of Kelly Brady in the table below.

Assessment Area	Kelly Brady's Findings
Head & Neck Sensory	
Neurologic	
Chest Respiratory	
Abdomen Gastrointestinal	
Lower Extremities Neurologic	

3. List interventions that the nurse caring for Kelly Brady will need to include in the plan of care.

4. When are antihypertensive medications traditionally administered to a patient who has gestational hypertension?

5. _____ Vasodilation in gestational hypertension results in proteinuria, hypertension, and edema. (True or False)

6. Match each sign or symptom below with its associated preeclampsia pathology. (*Note:* Some letters will be used more than once.)

Sign/Symptom	Pathology
_____ Blurred vision/blind spots	a. Generalized vasoconstriction
_____ Headache	b. Glomerular damage
_____ Epigastric or right upper quadrant abdominal pain	c. Retinal arteriolar spasms
_____ Hyperreflexia	d. Hepatic microemboli; liver damage
_____ Elevated blood pressure	e. Cortical brain spasms
_____ Proteinuria/oliguria	

7. When blood pressure levels warrant the management of hypertensive conditions of pregnancy medications may be administered. What classifications of medications may be used?

Exercise 3

Virtual Hospital Activity

30 minutes

- Sign in to work at Pacific View Regional Hospital on the Obstetrics Floor for Period of Care 3. (*Note:* If you are already in the virtual hospital from a previous exercise, click on **Leave the Floor** and then on **Restart the Program** to get to the sign-in window.)
- From the Patient List, select Kelly Brady (Room 203).
- Click on **Go to Nurses' Station**.

Read about HELLP syndrome in your textbook.

1. What is the rationale for Kelly Brady's AST measurement and platelet count drawn at 1230 on Wednesday?

- Click on **Chart** and then on **203**.
- Click on the **Laboratory Reports** tab and scroll down to review the results for Wednesday 1230.

2. Complete the table below based on your review of the Laboratory Reports and your textbook reading.

Test	Wednesday 1230 Result	Value in HELLP
Platelet count		
AST		

- Click on **Return to Nurses' Station** and then on **Patient List**.
- Click on **Get Report** for Kelly Brady.

3. Why has Kelly Brady been transferred to Labor and Delivery?

4. What do the letters in HELLP syndrome stand for?

- Click on **Return to Nurses' Station**.
- Click on **Chart** and then on **203**.
- Click on the **Physician's Notes** tab and review the note for Wednesday 1530. (*Note:* If the note you wish to see is not listed, this means you have not yet reached the correct virtual time to view that note. Click on the fast-forward icon within the virtual clock to advance the time by 2-minute intervals. Then click again on **Chart** and **203** to refresh the screen.)

5. HELLP syndrome is a variant of what condition?

6. What is the physician's plan of care for Kelly Brady in light of the HELLP syndrome diagnosis?

You will be the nurse caring for Kelly Brady after her surgery. She will be receiving magnesium sulfate during the postoperative period. Read about this medication in your textbook.

7. All of the assessments/interventions listed below are part of routine nursing care for a patient with severe preeclampsia. Place an X beside each of the activities performed specifically to assess for magnesium toxicity. Select all that apply.

_____   Measuring/recording urine output

_____   Measuring proteinuria using urine dipstick

_____   Monitoring liver enzyme levels and platelet count

_____   Monitoring for headache, visual disturbances, and epigastric pain

_____   Assessing for decreased level of consciousness

_____   Assessing DTRs

_____   Weighing daily to assess for edema

_____   Monitoring vital signs, especially respiratory rate

_____   Dimming room lights and maintaining a quiet environment

8. As the nurse caring for Kelly Brady during the administration of magnesium sulfate, you must have which antidote on hand?
   a. Calcium gluconate
   b. Narcan
   c. Diphenhydramine
   d. Benadryl

9. When monitoring Kelly Brady's serum magnesium levels, what level is considered therapeutic?
   a. 2-4 mg/dL
   b. 3-7 mg/dL
   c. 4-8 mg/dL
   d. 5-10 mg/dL

Nursing Care of Women with Complications During Pregnancy: Gestational Diabetes Mellitus

---

Reading Assignment: Nursing Care of Women with Complications During Pregnancy (Chapter 5)

Patient: Stacey Crider, Obstetrics Floor, Room 202

Objectives:

1. Identify appropriate interventions for controlling hyperglycemia in a patient with gestational diabetes mellitus (GDM).
2. Correctly administer insulin to a patient with GDM.
3. Plan and evaluate essential patient teaching for a patient with GDM.

In this lesson you will describe, plan, and evaluate the care of a patient with GDM.

Exercise 1

Virtual Hospital Activity

30 minutes

- Sign in to work at Pacific View Regional Hospital on the Obstetrics Floor for Period of Care 2. (*Note:* If you are already in the virtual hospital from a previous exercise, click on **Leave the Floor** and then on **Restart the Program** to get to the sign-in window.)
- From the Patient List, select Stacey Crider (Room 202).
- Click on **Go to Nurses' Station**.
- Click on **Chart** and then on **202**.
- Click on the **History and Physical** tab and review the information given.

1. Which hormones affect the actions of insulin during the pregnancy? Select all that apply.

   _____ Estrogen

   _____ Progesterone

   _____ Insulinase

   _____ Human gonadotropic hormone

   _____ Prolactin

   _____ Relaxin

2. Which complications of pregnancy may occur as a result of diabetes? Select all that apply.

   _____ Urinary tract infections

   _____ Oligohydramnios

   _____ Gestational hypertension

   _____ Birth canal injuries

   _____ Intrauterine growth restriction

   _____ Neonatal hyperbilirubinemia and jaundice

   _____ Fetal hyperglycemia

3. At what point in the gestational period is routine screening for gestational diabetes performed?
   a. 12-16 weeks
   b. 16-20 weeks
   c. 20-24 weeks
   d. 24-28 weeks

4. When was Stacey Crider's GDM diagnosed? How has it been managed so far?

5. List the risk factors for GDM.

• Click on **Nursing Admission** and **History and Physical** and review the information given.

6. Review the History and Physical and Nursing Admission tabs of Stacey Crider's chart. What risk factors for the development of gestational diabetes mellitus are noted?

7. What does Stacey Crider's physician suspect is the cause of her poorly controlled blood glucose levels? (*Hint:* See the physician's impression within her History and Physical.)

• Click on the **Physician's Orders** tab.

8. Review Stacey Crider's admission orders and list the orders that are related to her GDM.

9. Why are most oral hypoglycemic agents avoided during the prenatal period?

- Click on **Return to Nurses' Station**.
- Click on the **Drug** icon in the lower left corner of the screen.
- Use the search box or scroll down the list of medications to find betamethasone.

10. On admission, Stacey Crider was in preterm labor. This was treated with magnesium sulfate tocolysis. She was also given a course of betamethasone. What impact can betamethasone administration have on her gestational diabetes mellitus?

- Click on **Return to Nurses' Station**.
- Click on **Chart** and then on **202**.
- Click on the **Physician's Notes** tab and review the note for Tuesday at 0700.

11. How does Stacey Crider's physician plan to deal with these potential medication effects?

- Click on **Return to Nurses' Station** and then on **202** at the bottom of the screen.
- Click on **Patient Care** and then on **Nurse-Client Interactions**.
- Select and view the video titled **1115: Teaching—Diet, Infection**. (*Note:* Check the virtual clock to see whether enough time has elapsed. You can use the fast-forward feature to advance the time by 2-minute intervals if the video is not yet available. Then click again on **Patient Care** and **Nurse-Client Interactions** to refresh the screen.)

12. Stacey Crider's other admission diagnosis is bacterial vaginosis (BV). What is the relationship between the BV infection and her GDM?

Exercise 2

Virtual Hospital Activity

15 minutes

- Sign in to work at Pacific View Regional Hospital on the Obstetrics Floor for Period of Care 1. (*Note:* If you are already in the virtual hospital from a previous exercise, click on **Leave the Floor** and then on **Restart the Program** to get to the sign-in window.)
- From the Patient List, select Stacey Crider (Room 202).
- Click on **Go to Nurses' Station**.
- Click on the **Drug** icon in the lower left corner of the screen.
- Stacey Crider needs her insulin so that she can eat breakfast. She receives lispro insulin before each meal and NPH insulin at bedtime. Read about the differences in these two types of insulin in the Drug Guide.

1. Based on the Drug Guide, complete the table below.

Type of Insulin	Onset of Action	Peak	Duration
Lispro			
NPH			

- Click on **Return to Nurses' Station**.
- Click on **EPR** and then on **Login**.
- Select **202** from the Patient drop-down menu and select **Vital Signs** from the Category drop-down menu.
- Review the vital sign assessment for Wednesday at 0700.

2. What is Stacey Crider's blood glucose?

- Click on **Exit EPR**.
- Click on **MAR** and then on **202**.

3. What is Stacey Crider's prescribed insulin dosage?

- Click on **Return to Nurses' Station**.
- Click on **Chart** and then on **202**.
- Click on the **Physician's Orders** tab and review the orders for Tuesday at 1900.

4. How much insulin should Stacey Crider receive? Why?

- Click on **Return to Nurses' Station**.
- Click on **Medication Room**.
- Click on **Unit Dosage** and then on drawer **202**.
- Select **Insulin Lispro**; then click on **Put Medication on Tray**.
- Click on **Close Drawer** and then on **View Medication Room**.
- Click on **Preparation** and then on **Prepare** (next to Insulin Lispro).
- Follow the prompts to complete preparation of Stacey Crider's lispro insulin dose.
- Click on **Return to Medication Room**.

You are almost ready to give Stacey Crider's insulin injection. However, before you do . . .

5. Consider lispro insulin's rapid onset of action. What else should you check before giving Stacey Crider her injection?

Now you're ready!

- Click on **202** at the bottom of the screen to return to the patient's room.
- Inside the room, click on **Check Armband**.
- Click on **Patient Care** and then on **Medication Administration**.
- Insulin Lispro should be listed as a medication set aside for Stacey Crider.
- Click on the arrow next to Select and choose **Administer** from the drop-down menu.
- Follow the prompts to administer Stacey Crider's insulin injection. Document the injection in the MAR.
- Click on **Leave the Floor**; then click on **Look at Your Preceptor's Evaluation**.
- Click on **Medication Scorecard**. How did you do?
- Click on **Return to Evaluations** and then on **Return to Menu**.

Exercise 3

Virtual Hospital Activity

30 minutes

- Sign in to work at Pacific View Regional Hospital on the Obstetrics Floor for Period of Care 3. (*Note:* If you are already in the virtual hospital from a previous exercise, click on **Leave the Floor** and then on **Restart the Program** to get to the sign-in window.)
- From the Patient List, select Stacey Crider (Room 202).
- Click on **Go to Nurses' Station**.
- Click on **Chart** and then on **202**.
- Click on the **Patient Education** tab.

Stacey Crider will probably be discharged soon. Review her Patient Education record to determine her learning needs in relation to GDM.

1. List the educational goals for Stacey Crider regarding GDM.

2. Which of Stacey Crider's educational goals would apply to all women with GDM?

3. Which of Stacey Crider's educational goals would not apply to all women with GDM? Support your answer.

- Click on the **Nurse's Notes** tab and review the note for 0600 Wednesday.

4. How did the nurse describe Stacey Crider's ability to give her own insulin injection at that time?

- Click again on **Patient Education**.

5. What teaching has already been done with this patient on Wednesday in regard to GDM?

- Click on **Nurse's Notes** and scroll to the note for 1200 Wednesday.

6. Do you think today's initial teaching on insulin administration was effective? Support your answer using objective documentation from the Nurse's Notes.

7. Stacey Crider needs to know all of the following information. Which topic(s) would you choose to cover with her during this period of care? (*Hint:* Review the Patient Education and Nurse's Notes in her chart.) Select all that apply.

_____ Verbalize appropriate food choices and portions

_____ Demonstrate good technique when administering insulin

_____ Demonstrate good technique with self-monitoring of blood glucose

_____ Recognize hyper- and hypoglycemia and how to treat each

8. Give a rationale for the choice(s) you made in the previous question

9. Which topic do you think Stacey Crider would most likely choose to work on during this period of care?
   a. Verbalize appropriate food choices and portions
   b. Demonstrate good technique when administering insulin
   c. Demonstrate good technique with self-monitoring of blood glucose
   d. Recognize hyper- and hypoglycemia and how to treat each

10. Give a rationale for the choice you made in the previous question.

11. Which statement concerning insulin needs in pregnancy is most correct?
    a. Insulin needs during the pregnancy will gradually decrease.
    b. Insulin needs during pregnancy remain at a constant level.
    c. Insulin needs may decrease in the last few weeks of pregnancy.
    d. Insulin needs are greatest in the first trimester.

12. Stacey Crider has a significant risk for developing glucose intolerance later in life. What advice would you give Stacey Crider to reduce this risk?

13. Could Stacey Crider's GDM affect her baby after birth? Explain.

Nursing Care of Women with Complications During Pregnancy: Cardiac and Lupus

Reading Assignment: Nursing Care of Women with Complications During Pregnancy (Chapter 5)

Patients: Maggie Gardner, Obstetrics Floor, Room 204
Gabriela Valenzuela, Obstetrics Floor, Room 205

Objectives:

1. Identify appropriate interventions for managing selected medical-surgical problems in pregnancy.
2. Plan and evaluate essential patient education during the acute phase of diagnosis.

Exercise 1

Virtual Hospital Activity

10 minutes

- Sign in to work at Pacific View Regional Hospital on the Obstetrics Floor for Period of Care 1. (*Note:* If you are already in the virtual hospital from a previous exercise, click on **Leave the Floor** and then on **Restart the Program** to get to the sign-in window.)
- From the Patient List, select Gabriela Valenzuela (Room 205).
- Click on **Go to Nurses' Station**.
- Click on **Chart** and then on **205** to view Gabriela Valenzuela's chart.
- Click on the **History and Physical** tab and review the information given.

Review cardiac problems during pregnancy in your textbook.

1. After reviewing the History and Physical for Gabriela Valenzuela, what does the physician note as her cardiac problem?

2. A pregnant woman with cardiac disease is placed at a higher risk for additional complications because of which pregnancy-related phenomena? Select all that apply.

_____ Elevations in blood pressure in the second and third trimesters

_____ Increase in heart rate

_____ Increase in blood volume

_____ Increase in body temperature

_____ Increase in cardiac output

3. Congestive heart failure is a complication for the pregnant woman with heart disease. What are clinical manifestations associated with congestive heart failure? Select all that apply.

_____ Bradycardia

_____ Orthopnea

_____ Persistent cough

_____ Pitting edema

_____ Moist lung fields

4. According to the History and Physical, what cardiac symptoms does Gabriela Valenzuela exhibit now that she is pregnant?

5. What are Gabriela Valenzuela's vital signs? Are there any significant abnormalities noted?

6. What abnormal assessment finding is noted in the History and Physical that would be associated with Gabriela Valenzuela's cardiac disorder?

7. When monitoring Gabriela Valenzuela's fetus, what manifestations may indicate complications related to a worsening of the mother's cardiac status?
   a. Fetal bradycardia
   b. Fetal tachycardia
   c. Increasing fetal size, greater than anticipated for gestational age
   d. Increasing fetal temperature

8. _____ Cesarean section is the preferred type of delivery for the mother with cardiac disease. (True or False)

9. When considering the risks to Gabriela Valenzuela as a result of her cardiac condition, what two gestational periods are problematic?

   _____ First trimester

   _____ Second trimester

   _____ Third trimester

   _____ Labor

   _____ Early postpartum

10. Provide a rationale for your answer to the previous question.

Exercise 2

Virtual Hospital Activity

30 minutes

- Sign in to work at Pacific View Regional Hospital on the Obstetrics Floor for Period of Care 2. (*Note:* If you are already in the virtual hospital from a previous exercise, click on **Leave the Floor** and then on **Restart the Program** to get to the sign-in window.)
- From the Patient List, select Maggie Gardner (Room 204).
- Click on **Go to Nurses' Station**.
- Click on **Chart** and then on **204** to view Maggie Gardner's chart.
- Click on the **History and Physical** tab and review the information given.

Autoimmune disorders encompass a wide variety of disorders that can be disruptive to the pregnancy process. Maggie Gardner has been admitted to rule out lupus. The following questions will explore the various aspects of this autoimmune disorder. You may want to review information from a medical-surgical textbook regarding this disease.

1. What information in Maggie Gardner's History and Physical would correlate to a diagnosis of systemic lupus erythematosus (SLE)?

- Click on **Return to Nurses' Station** and then on **204** at the bottom of the screen.
- Click on **Patient Care** and complete a head-to-toe assessment of Maggie Gardner by clicking on the various body systems (yellow buttons) and body system subcategories (green buttons).

2. List at least four abnormal findings related to Maggie Gardner's potential diagnosis.

- Click on **Chart** and then on **204** to view Maggie Gardner's chart.
- Click on the **Patient Education** tab and review the information given.

3. Based on your physical assessment of Maggie Gardner, the information presented in the Patient Education section of the chart, and the fact that this is a new diagnosis for the patient, list at least three areas of teaching that need to be covered at this time.

Exercise 3

Virtual Hospital Activity

30 minutes

- Sign in to work at Pacific View Regional Hospital on the Obstetrics Floor for Period of Care 3. (*Note:* If you are already in the virtual hospital from a previous exercise, click on **Leave the Floor** and then on **Restart the Program** to get to the sign-in window.)
- From the Patient List, select Maggie Gardner (Room 204).
- Click on **Go to Nurses' Station**.
- Click on **Chart** and then on **204** to view Maggie Gardner's chart.
- Click on the **Consultations** tab review the Rheumatology Consult.

1. List four things that the rheumatologist notes in his impressions regarding specific findings associated with a diagnosis of SLE.

2. What is the rheumatologist's plan regarding laboratory/diagnostics to gain a definitive diagnosis?

3. According to the Rheumatology Consult, what is the plan regarding medications (immediate need)?

- Click on the **Diagnostic Reports** tab and review the information given.

4. Maggie Gardner had an ultrasound done before the consult with the rheumatologist. What were the findings in regard to SLE? What were the follow-up recommendations? (*Hint:* See Impression section.)

- Click on **Return to Nurses' Station**.
- Click on the **Drug** icon in the lower left corner of the screen.
- Use the search box or scroll down the list of medications to find and review prednisone.

5. When providing teaching about the use of prednisone, the nurse should include what information? Select all that apply.

    _____ Prednisone therapy is associated with increased levels of fatigue.

    _____ The onset of fever, muscle aches, and sore throat is a common side effect.

    _____ Limit caffeine during prednisone therapy.

    _____ Prednisone use may be associated with mood swings, ranging from euphoria to depression.

    _____ Do not abruptly discontinue drug therapy without consulting physician.

6. The physician has prescribed prednisone therapy. Which statement best describes its purpose?
    a. Reduces susceptibility to infection
    b. Reduces the body's inflammatory response
    c. Enhances the body's use of acetylcholine
    d. Stimulates lung development in the fetus

- Click on **Return to Nurse's Station** and then on **204** at the bottom of the screen.
- Click on **Patient Care** and then on **Nurse-Client Interactions**.
- Select and view the video titled **1530: Disease Management**. (*Note:* Check the virtual clock to see whether enough time has elapsed. You can use the fast-forward feature to advance the time by 2-minute intervals if the video is not yet available. Then click again on **Patient Care** and **Nurse-Client Interactions** to refresh the screen.)

7. During this video, the nurse provides Maggie Gardner with information regarding her disease. What two things does the nurse note that are important aspects of disease management during pregnancy?

8. What medication ordered by the rheumatologist will assist in the blood flow to the placenta? How does this medication achieve this effect?

9. What key component does the nurse identify for Maggie Gardner that will assist in maintaining a healthy pregnancy?

10. What does Maggie Gardner give as her reason for not keeping previous appointments? (*Hint:* See the Nursing Admission in her chart.)

Exercise 4

Virtual Hospital Activity

10 minutes

- Sign in to work at Pacific View Regional Hospital on the Obstetrics Floor for Period of Care 4. (*Note:* If you are already in the virtual hospital from a previous exercise, click on **Leave the Floor** and then on **Restart the Program** to get to the sign-in window. Remember that you cannot perform patient care during Period of Care 4. You may, however, view patient records for all periods of care.)
- Click on **Chart** and then on **204** to view Maggie Gardner's chart.
- Click on the **Laboratory Reports** tab and review the results.

1. What are the findings for each of the laboratory tests that were ordered for Maggie Gardner in Period of Care 2?

Laboratory Test	Maggie Gardner's Results
C3	
C4	
CH50	
RPR	
ANA titer	
Anticardiolipin	
Anti-sm, anti-DNA, anti-SSA	
Anti-SSB	
Anti-RVV, antiphospholipid	

- Click on the **Nurse's Notes** tab and review the information given.

2. Maggie Gardner has been provided with education regarding various aspects of her disease process, testing, and hospital procedures. Based on your review of the Nurse's Notes for Wednesday, list what she has been specifically taught during the four periods of care today. (*Note:* Include the time and instruction provided.)

3. Using NANDA nursing diagnosis wording and format, write three possible nursing diagnoses for Maggie Gardner.

- Click on the **Consultations** tab and review the Rheumatology Consult and the Pastoral Consult.

4. SLE requires long-term management as patients experience remissions and exacerbations. What did the rheumatologist do to establish the long-term relationship with Maggie Gardner necessary to ensure a healthy outcome?

5. To what does Maggie Gardner attribute her inability to have a child?

6. When working with Maggie Gardner, what interventions can the nurse utilize to work through the grieving process with the patient? Select all that apply.

_____ Explain that each pregnancy is different and that the baby she is carrying needs for her to focus on her own care.

_____ Offer to contact the hospital chaplain.

_____ Offer emotional support.

_____ Encourage her to verbalize her feelings.

7. Grief is a very individualized emotion. List four common reactions to grieving.

8. Compare Maggie Gardner's History and Physical with what typically happens during the reorganization phase. What correlation do you see?

Nursing Care of Women with Complications During Pregnancy: Substance Abuse/Battering

Reading Assignment: Nursing Care of Women with Complications During Pregnancy (Chapter 5)

Patients: Dorothy Grant, Obstetrics Floor, Room 201
Laura Wilson, Obstetrics Floor, Room 206

Objectives:

1. Assess and plan care for a substance-abusing woman with a term pregnancy.
2. Discuss the statistics related to battering.
3. List characteristics of battered women.
4. Explore the myths and facts regarding battering.
5. Identify the nurse's role in regard to battered women.

Exercise 1

Virtual Hospital Activity

30 minutes

- Sign in to work at Pacific View Regional Hospital on the Obstetrics Floor for Period of Care 2. (*Note:* If you are already in the virtual hospital from a previous exercise, click on **Leave the Floor** and then on **Restart the Program** to get to the sign-in window.)
- From the Patient List, select Laura Wilson (Room 206).
- Click on **Go to Nurses' Station**.
- Click on **Chart** and then on **206** to view Laura Wilson's chart.
- Click on the **Nursing Admission** tab and review the information given.

1. Complete the table below with information regarding Laura Wilson's use of alcohol and recreational drugs. (*Hint:* See page 4 of the Nursing Admission.)

Substance	Reported Use
Tobacco	
Alcohol	
Marijuana	
Crack cocaine	

Read about tobacco, alcohol, marijuana, and cocaine in the Substance Abuse section in your textbook.

2. Laura Wilson's Nursing Admission assessment indicates that she has used cocaine. Which complication is linked to the use of this substance?
   a. Placental perfusion abnormalities
   b. Addiction of the newborn
   c. Hypotension
   d. Low birth weight

3. Laura Wilson's Nursing Assessment indicates that she smokes cigarettes. Which complications are associated with this practice? Select all that apply.

   _____ Low birth weight

   _____ Newborn nicotine addiction

   _____ Placental perfusion abnormalities

   _____ Fetal anomalies

   _____ Hyperemesis

4. Mental retardation in children has been linked to which behavior?
   a. Tobacco use in pregnancy
   b. Alcohol use in pregnancy
   c. Marijuana use in pregnancy
   d. Cocaine use in pregnancy

- Click on **Return to Nurses' Station** and then on **206** at the bottom of the screen.
- Click on **Patient Care** and then on **Nurse-Client Interactions**.
- Select and view the video titled **1115: Teaching—Effects of Drug Use**. (*Note:* Check the virtual clock to see whether enough time has elapsed. You can use the fast-forward feature to advance the time by 2-minute intervals if the video is not yet available. Then click again on **Patient Care** and **Nurse-Client Interactions** to refresh the screen.)

5. Does Laura Wilson consider herself to be addicted? Support your answer with comments from the video interaction.

6. How does Laura Wilson think her drug use will affect the baby?

7. According to the nurse in the video, how might Laura Wilson's drug use affect the baby?

8. Assume that you are the nurse caring for Laura Wilson today. Which interventions dealing with her drug use would be most appropriate at this time? Select all that apply.

   _____ Talking with Laura Wilson in a manner that conveys caring and concern

   _____ Urging Laura Wilson to begin a drug treatment program today

   _____ Explaining to Laura Wilson that she may lose custody of her baby if her drug use continues

   _____ Involving other members of the health care team in Laura Wilson's care

9. After birth, Laura Wilson's baby will need to be closely assessed for fetal alcohol syndrome. Which manifestations may be associated with this condition? Select all that apply.

   _____ Microcephaly

   _____ Thickened upper lip

   _____ Sharp facial features

   _____ Flat nasal bridge

   _____ Short palpebral (eye) fissures

Exercise 2

Virtual Hospital Activity

30 minutes

Review the characteristics of battered women found in your textbook.

1. Battering occurs in _____ ethnic groups and at _____ social levels.

• Sign in to work at Pacific View Regional Hospital on the Obstetrics Floor for Period of Care 1. (*Note:* If you are already in the virtual hospital from a previous exercise, click on **Leave the Floor** and then on **Restart the Program** to get to the sign-in window.)
• From the Patient List, select Dorothy Grant (Room 201).
• Click on **Go to Nurses' Station**.
• Click on **Chart** and then on **201** to view Dorothy Grant's chart.
• Click on the **Nursing Admission** tab and review Dorothy Grant's perspective of her abusive relationship.

2. What is the reality of Dorothy Grant's situation (as evidenced in the Nursing Admission), and how does that correlate with the textbook reading?

• Click on **Return to Nurses' Station** and then on **201** at the bottom of the screen.
• Click on **Patient Care** and then on **Nurse-Client Interactions**.
• Select and view the video titled **0810: Monitoring/Patient Support**. (*Note:* Check the virtual clock to see whether enough time has elapsed. You can use the fast-forward feature to advance the time by 2-minute intervals if the video is not yet available. Then click again on **Patient Care** and **Nurse-Client Interactions** to refresh the screen.)

3. What does Dorothy Grant say that she should do to help prevent the violence?

4. What are the greatest concerns for Dorothy Grant at this time?

- Click on **Chart** and then on **201**.
- Click on the **History and Physical** and **Nursing Admission** tabs and review the information given.

5. Battered women share many characteristics. Compare the following list of characteristics from your textbook with Dorothy Grant's situation. For each characteristic listed, write Yes or No to indicate whether or not it applies to Dorothy Grant. For all Yes answers, provide a rationale to explain how that characteristic applies to her. (*Hint:* You may want to watch the 0810 video again in addition to reviewing the History and Physical and Nursing Admission)

Textbook Characteristics of Battered Women	If/How Each Characteristic Applies to Dorothy Grant
Financially dependent	
Few resources/support systems	
Blame themselves for what has taken place	
State they are not "good enough"	
Bonding occurs out of fear and helplessness	
Low self-esteem	
History of domestic violence in their family	
Fear societal rejection	
Strong nurturing, yielding personality	

Textbook Characteristics of Battered Women	If/How Each Characteristic Applies to Dorothy Grant
Tolerate control from others easily	
Attempt to avoid arousing anger in the abuser	
Deliberate/repeated physical or sexual assault	

6. What is the time period of greatest danger for the battered woman?

Let's jump ahead in virtual time to review some records that are not available until later in the day.

- Click on **Return to Room 201**; then click on **Leave the Floor** and **Restart the Program** to return to the sign-in window.
- Sign in to work at Pacific View Regional Hospital on the Obstetrics Floor for Period of Care 3.
- From the Patient List, select Dorothy Grant (Room 201).
- Click on **Go to Nurses' Station**.
- Click on **Chart** and then on **201** to view Dorothy Grant's chart.
- Click on the **Consultations** tab and review the Psychiatric Consult and Social Work Consult.

7. According to these consultations, Dorothy Grant has several options. What do the social worker and psychiatric health care provider suggest to her or assist her with?

8. Indicate whether each statement is true or false.

a. _____ Battering often escalates or begins during pregnancy.

b. _____ Dorothy Grant's husband blames her for the pregnancy.

c. _____ Dorothy Grant stays in the relationship because she likes to be beaten and deliberately provokes the attacks on occasion.

Exercise 3

Virtual Hospital Activity

15 minutes

- Sign in to work at Pacific View Regional Hospital on the Obstetrics Floor for Period of Care 4. (*Note:* If you are already in the virtual hospital from a previous exercise, click on **Leave the Floor** and then on **Restart the Program** to get to the sign-in window. Remember that you cannot perform patient care during Period of Care 4. You may, however, view patient records for all periods of care.)
- Click on **Kardex** and then on **201** to review Dorothy Grant's Kardex.

1. What action was initiated on Wednesday to protect Dorothy Grant from her husband?

2. What nursing care plan diagnoses are appropriate for Dorothy Grant's current life situation?

3. Members of what other disciplines have been contacted or consulted and will ensure continuity of care for Dorothy Grant as it relates to her abuse?

4. What is your responsibility, as a nurse, for reporting battering?

5. What resources are available in your area for women who are experiencing battering?

Nursing Management of Pain During Labor and Birth

Reading Assignment: Nursing Management of Pain During Labor and Birth (Chapter 7)

Patients: Kelly Brady, Obstetrics Floor, Room 203
Gabriela Valenzuela, Obstetrics Floor, Room 205
Laura Wilson, Obstetrics Floor, Room 206

Objectives:

1. Compare true and false labor.
2. Review the stages or phases of labor.
3. Assess and identify factors that influence pain perception.
4. Describe selected nonpharmacological and pharmacological measures for pain management during labor and birth.

In this lesson you will compare and contrast the pain management strategies used with three patients during labor and birth.

Exercise 1

Virtual Hospital Activity

15 minutes

- Sign in to work at Pacific View Regional Hospital on the Obstetrics Floor for Period of Care 1. (*Note:* If you are already in the virtual hospital from a previous exercise, click on **Leave the Floor** and then on **Restart the Program** to get to the sign-in window.)
- From the Patient List, select Laura Wilson (Room 206).
- Click on **Get Report** and read the Clinical Report.

1. What is Laura Wilson's condition, according to the Clinical Report?

- Click on **Go to Nurses' Station** and then on **206** at the bottom of the screen.
- Inside the patient's room, read the Initial Observations.

2. What is your impression of Laura Wilson's condition?

- Click on **Patient Care** and then on **Nurse-Client Interactions**.
- Select and view the video titled **0730: Patient Assessment**. (*Note:* Check the virtual clock to see whether enough time has elapsed. You can use the fast-forward feature to advance the time by 2-minute intervals if the video is not yet available. Then click again on **Patient Care** and **Nurse-Client Interactions** to refresh the screen.)

3. What is Laura Wilson's assessment of her current condition? How does this compare with the information you received from the Clinical Report and the Initial Observations summary?

- Click on **Chart** and then on **206** to view Laura Wilson's chart.
- Click on the **Nursing Admission** tab and review the information given.

4. List Laura Wilson's admission diagnoses. (*Hint:* See page 1 of the Nursing Admission form.)

5. Which factor in Laura Wilson's history will likely have the greatest impact on the management of her pain?
   a. HIV-positive status
   b. History of illegal drug use
   c. Vomiting and diarrhea
   d. Unmarried

6. Think about the following questions and then discuss your ideas with your classmates: Do your personal values and beliefs contribute to your perception of Laura Wilson's behavior? If so, how? What nursing interventions might help to overcome your personal biases when dealing with Laura Wilson?

Exercise 2

Virtual Hospital Activity

45 minutes

Review the sections on skin stimulation and breathing techniques in your textbook.

1. A pregnant woman reports having read of a childbirth technique that promotes slow abdominal breathing and relaxation. The nurse correctly recognizes that this method is known as the _____ method.
   a. Dick-Read
   b. Lamaze
   c. Bradley
   d. Effleurage training

2. Which technique is more often associated with prepared childbirth?
   a. Effleurage
   b. Controlled breathing
   c. Paced breathing
   d. Distraction

- Sign in to work at Pacific View Regional Hospital on the Obstetrics Floor for Period of Care 2. (*Note:* If you are already in the virtual hospital from a previous exercise, click on **Leave the Floor** and then on **Restart the Program** to get to the sign-in window.)
- From the Patient List, select Gabriela Valenzuela (Room 205).
- Click on **Get Report** and read the Clinical Report.

Review the section on systemic analgesia in your textbook.

3. What is Gabriela Valenzuela's current labor assessment? Include information about her degree of dilation, effacement, and contractions.

4. Review the signs and symptoms listed below. Indicate whether they are signs of true labor or false labor.

Sign/Symptom	True or False Labor?
_____ Discomfort is in abdomen.	a. True labor
_____ Bloody show is present.	b. False labor
_____ Contractions become progressively stronger.	
_____ May initially feel like menstrual cramps.	
_____ Walking relieves contraction pain.	
_____ Contractions become more intense.	

5. What are Gabriela Valenzuela's fetal heart tones? Are they within normal range?

6. What phase or stage of labor is Gabriela Valenzuela in?
   a. Latent phase
   b. Active phase
   c. Transition phase
   d. Stage 2

- Click on **Go to Nurses' Station** and then on **205** at the bottom of the screen.
- Click on **Patient Care** and then on **Nurse-Client Interactions**.
- Select and view the video titled **1140: Intervention—Bleeding, Comfort**. (*Note:* Check the virtual clock to see whether enough time has elapsed. You can use the fast-forward feature to advance the time by 2-minute intervals if the video is not yet available. Then click again on **Patient Care** and **Nurse-Client Interactions** to refresh the screen.)
- Click on **Chart** and then on **205** to view Gabriela Valenzuela's chart.
- Click on the **Nurse's Notes** tab and review the entry for 1140 on Wednesday.

7. How is Gabriela Valenzuela tolerating labor at this time?

8. What pain interventions is the nurse implementing at this time?

9. What is the action of fentanyl?

Let's begin the process of preparing and administering Gabriela Valenzuela's fentanyl dose.

- Click on **Return to Room 205** and then on **Medication Room**.
- Click on **MAR** and then on **205**.
- Review the PRN medication administration record for Wednesday.

10. What is the ordered dose of fentanyl?

- Click on **Return to Room 205**.
- Click on **Medication Room**.
- Click on **Automated System** and then on **Login**.
- Select **Gabriela Valenzuela** and then select **Automated System Drawer (A-F)**.
- Click on **Open Drawer**.
- Select **Fentanyl citrate**; then click on **Put Medication on Tray**.
- Click on **Close Drawer**.
- Click on **View Medication Room** and then on **Preparation**.
- Click on **Prepare** and follow the Preparation Wizard prompts.
- Click on **Return to Medication Room** and then on **205** at the bottom of the screen to go to the patient's room.

11. What additional assessments must be completed before you give Gabriela Valenzuela's medication?

12. Why is it important to check Gabriela Valenzuela's respirations before giving the dose of fentanyl?

13. What safety precautions should be in effect for Gabriela Valenzuela after she receives this dose of fentanyl?

- Click on **Patient Care** and then on **Medication Administration**.
- Click on **Review Your Medications** and then on the **Prepared** tab to verify the accuracy of your preparation.
- Click on **Return to Room 205**.
- Click on the arrow next to Select and choose **Administer** from the drop-down menu.
- Follow the Administration Wizard prompts to administer Gabriela Valenzuela's fentanyl dose. Click **Yes** when asked whether to document this administration in the MAR.
- Click on **Patient Care** and then on **Nurse-Client Interactions**.
- Select and view the video titled **1155: Evaluation—Comfort Measures**. (*Note:* Check the virtual clock to see whether enough time has elapsed. You can use the fast-forward feature to advance the time by 2-minute intervals if the video is not yet available. Then click again on **Patient Care** and **Nurse-Client Interactions** to refresh the screen.)

14. Based on this video interaction, how effective were the nursing interventions that you identified in question 8?

15. Gabriela Valenzuela is experiencing _____. _____

_____ is responsible for the dizziness, as well as other side effects,

including _____ _____ and numbness around the

_____ and _____.

16. What interventions does the nurse suggest to deal with the above problem that Gabriela Valenzuela is experiencing? List other interventions as described in your textbook.

At the end of the 1155 video, Gabriela Valenzuela states that she "doesn't want any needles" in her back. Learn more about this procedure by reading the Epidural Analgesia/Anesthesia section in your textbook.

17. What could you tell Gabriela Valenzuela to help her make an informed decision about anesthesia for labor? In the table below, list advantages and disadvantages of epidural anesthesia.

Advantages	Disadvantages

Let's see how you did preparing and administering the patient's medication.

- Click on **Leave the Floor** then on **Look at Your Preceptor's Evaluation**.
- Click on **Medication Scorecard** and review the evaluation. How did you do?
- Click on **Return to Evaluations** and then on **Return to Menu**.

Exercise 3

Virtual Hospital Activity

15 minutes

Read the General Anesthesia section on page 169 in your textbook.

- Sign in to work at Pacific View Regional Hospital on the Obstetrics Floor for Period of Care 4. (*Note:* If you are already in the virtual hospital from a previous exercise, click on **Leave the Floor** and then on **Restart the Program** to get to the sign-in window. Remember that you cannot perform patient care during Period of Care 4. You may, however, view patient records for all periods of care.)
- Click on **Chart** and then on **203** to view Kelly Brady's chart.
- Click on the **Nurse's Notes** tab and review the entry for 1730 on Wednesday.

1. Why does the anesthesiologist plan to use general anesthesia during Kelly Brady's cesarean section? (*Hint:* Read the Contraindications to Epidural Blocks section in your textbook.)

2. Why is Kelly Brady upset about receiving general anesthesia for her surgery?

- Click on the **Physician's Orders** tab and review the entry for Wednesday at 1540.

3. What preoperative medications have been ordered for Kelly Brady?

- Click on **Return to Nurses' Station**.
- Click on the **Drug** icon in the lower left corner of your screen.
- Review the medications that you listed in the previous answer.

4. All of the medications listed below are given preoperatively to help prevent aspiration pneumonia. Using information from the Drug Guide, match each medication below with the description of how it specifically works to prevent aspiration pneumonia.

	Medication		**Use in Preventing Pneumonia**
_____	Sodium citrate/citric acid (Bicitra)	a.	Decreases the production of gastric acid
_____	Metoclopramide (Reglan)	b.	Prevents nausea and vomiting; accelerates gastric emptying
_____	Ranitidine (Zantac)	c.	Neutralizes acidic stomach contents

5. How would you expect general anesthesia to affect Kelly Brady's baby? Why?

Nursing Care of Women with Complications During Labor and Birth

Reading Assignment: Nursing Care of Women with Complications During Labor and Birth
(Chapter 8)

Patients: Dorothy Grant, Obstetrics Floor, Room 201
Stacey Crider, Obstetrics Floor, Room 202
Kelly Brady, Obstetrics Floor, Room 203
Gabriela Valenzuela, Obstetrics Floor, Room 205

Objectives:

1. Assess and identify signs and symptoms present in the patient with preterm labor.
2. Describe appropriate nursing care for the patient in preterm labor.
3. Develop a birth plan to meet the needs of the preterm infant.

In this lesson you will compare and contrast the care of four patients, each of whom is treated for preterm labor and/or will deliver preterm infants.

Exercise 1

Virtual Hospital Activity

15 minutes

- Sign in to work at Pacific View Regional Hospital on the Obstetrics Floor for Period of Care 2. (*Note:* If you are already in the virtual hospital from a previous exercise, click on **Leave the Floor** and then on **Restart the Program** to get to the sign-in window.)
- From the Patient List, select Dorothy Grant (Room 201) and Gabriela Valenzuela (Room 205).
- Click on **Go to Nurses' Station**.
- Click on **Chart** and then on **201** to view Dorothy Grant's chart.
- Click on the **History and Physical** tab and review the information given.

1. Using the information found in the History and Physical section, complete the table below for Dorothy Grant.

Patient	Weeks Gestation	Reason for Admission
Dorothy Grant		
Gabriela Valenzuela		

- Click on **Return to Nurses' Station**.
- Click on **Chart** and then on **205** to view Gabriela Valenzuela's chart.
- Click on the **History and Physical** tab and review the information given.

2. Using the information found in the History and Physical section, complete the table above for Gabriela Valenzuela.

- Click on **Return to Nurses' Station** and then on **201** at the bottom of the screen to enter Dorothy Grant's room.
- Click on **Patient Care** and then on **Physical Assessment**.
- Click on **Pelvic** and then select the body system subcategories (green buttons) to perform a pelvic examination.

3. Complete the table below with the results of Dorothy Grant's initial cervical exam.

Patient	Time	Dilation	Effacement	Station
Dorothy Grant	0730			
Gabriela Valenzuela				

- Click on **Nurses' Station** and then on **205** at the bottom of the screen to enter Gabriela Valenzuela's room.
- Click on **Patient Care** and then on **Physical Assessment**.
- Click on **Pelvic** and then select the body system subcategories (green buttons) to perform a pelvic examination.

4. Record the results of Gabriela Valenzuela's initial cervical examination in the table above.

Read the Preterm Labor section in your textbook.

5. Which factors are considered to increase the risk for preterm labor? Select all that apply.

_____ Obesity

_____ Anemia

_____ Diabetes

_____ Hypertension

_____ Acute episodes of stress

_____ Inadequate prenatal care

_____ Poverty

_____ Low educational level

6. As of Wednesday at 0800, would you consider either or both of these patients to be in preterm labor? Give a rationale for your answer.

Read the Tocolytic Therapy section in your textbook to answer the following questions.

7. Match each medication below with its corresponding mechanism of action. Answers may be used more than once. (*Hint:* You may need to review the Drug Guide.)

Medication

_____ Magnesium sulfate

_____ Nifedipine (Procardia)

_____ Ritodrine (Yutopar)

_____ Terbutaline (Brethine)

_____ Indomethacin (Indocin)

Mechanism of Action

a. Inhibits calcium from entering smooth muscle cells, thus relaxing uterine contractions

b. Relaxes uterine smooth muscle as a result of stimulation of beta$_2$ receptors on uterine smooth muscle

c. Exact mechanism unclear, but promotes relaxation of smooth muscles

d. Suppresses preterm labor by blocking the production of prostaglandins

8. Which conditions and factors are contraindications to the use of tocolytic therapies? Select all that apply.

_____ Multifetal pregnancy

_____ Preeclampsia

_____ Hyperemesis

_____ Fetal demise

_____ Abruptio placentae

_____ Chorioamnionitis

Exercise 2

Virtual Hospital Activity

30 minutes

- Sign in to work at Pacific View Regional Hospital on the Obstetrics Floor for Period of Care 1. (*Note:* If you are already in the virtual hospital from a previous exercise, click on **Leave the Floor** and then on **Restart the Program** to get to the sign-in window.)
- From the Patient List, select Stacey Crider (Room 202).
- Click on **Get Report** and read the Clinical Report.

Stacey Crider was admitted yesterday in preterm labor and put on magnesium sulfate. Her other admission diagnoses were bacterial vaginosis and gestational diabetes with poorly controlled blood glucose levels.

1. What is Stacey Crider's current status in regard to preterm labor?

- Click on **Go to Nurses' Station**.
- Click on **Chart** and then on **202** to view Stacey Crider's chart.
- Click on the **Physician's Orders** tab and review the orders for Wednesday at 0715.

2. Which of these orders relates specifically to Stacey Crider's diagnosis of preterm labor?

- Now review the **Physician's Orders** for Wednesday at 0730.

3. What medication changes were ordered?

Read about terbutaline and nifedipine in the Tocolytic Therapy section in your textbook.

4. What adverse effects may have occurred if Stacey Crider had remained on terbutaline? (*Hint:* Consider Stacey Crider's gestational diabetes condition.)

* Click on **Return to Nurses' Station** and then on **202** at the bottom of the screen to enter Stacy Crider's room.
* Click on **Take Vital Signs**.

5. What are Stacey Crider's current vital signs? (*Note:* Answers will vary depending on the exact time you take the vital signs.)

    Temperature:

    Heart rate:

    Respirations:

    Blood pressure:

6. Which of the above parameters is the most crucial piece of information to obtain before giving Stacey Crider the ordered nifedipine dose?
    a. Temperature
    b. Heart rate
    c. Respirations
    d. Blood pressure

Like Dorothy Grant and Kelly Brady, Stacey Crider is also receiving betamethasone. Read the Speeding Fetal Lung Maturity section in your textbook on page 193.

7. All three of these patients are receiving antenatal glucocorticoid therapy. What is the anticipated impact of this medication on their condition?
    a. Increase placental perfusion
    b. Accelerate fetal lung maturity
    c. Further slow preterm labor contractions
    d. Reduce maternal anxiety

8. _____ The betamethasone therapy will enhance the effects of Stacey Crider's prescribed insulin. (True or False)

* Click on **MAR** and then on **202** to review Stacey Crider's MAR.

9. What is Stacey Crider's prescribed betamethasone dosage?

- Click on **Return to Room 202** and then on **Medication Room** at the bottom of the screen.
- Click on **Unit Dosage** and then on drawer **202**.
- Click on **Betamethasone** and then on **Put Medication on Tray**.
- Click on **Close Drawer**.
- Click on **View Medication Room** and then on **Preparation**.
- Click on **Prepare** (next to Betamethasone) and follow the Preparation Wizard prompts.
- Click on **Return to Medication Room**.
- Click on **202** at the bottom of the screen to return to Stacey Crider's room.
- Click on **Check Armband** and then on **Check Allergies**.
- Click on **Patient Care** and then on **Medication Administration**.
- Click on the arrow next to Select and choose **Administer**.
- Follow the Administration Wizard prompts. Check **Yes** to document this administration in the MAR.
- Click on **Leave the Floor**.
- Click on **Look at Your Preceptor's Evaluation** and then click on **Medication Scorecard**. How did you do?
- Click on **Return to Evaluations** and then on **Return to Menu**.

Exercise 3

Virtual Hospital Activity

30 minutes

- Sign in to work at Pacific View Regional Hospital on the Obstetrics Floor for Period of Care 4. (*Note:* If you are already in the virtual hospital from a previous exercise, click on **Leave the Floor** and then on **Restart the Program** to get to the sign-in window. Remember that you cannot perform patient care during Period of Care 4. You may, however, view patient records for all periods of care.)
- Click on **Chart** and then on **201** to view Dorothy Grant's chart.
- Click on the **Nurse's Notes** tab and review the note for Wednesday 1815.

1. What is the result of Dorothy Grant's cervical exam at this time?

- The **Nurse's Notes** for Wednesday 1840 states that Dorothy Grant is being prepped for delivery.

2. If you were the nurse caring for Dorothy Grant during delivery, what special preparations would you make to care for the baby immediately after birth?

- Click on **Return to Nurses' Station**.
- Click on **Chart** and then on **205** to view Gabriela Valenzuela's chart.
- Click on the **Physician's Notes** tab and review the note for Wednesday 0800.

3. What is the anticipated outcome of Gabriela Valenzuela's labor, according to this note?

- Review the **Physician's Notes** for Wednesday 1415 and 1455.

4. What preparations have been made during the day for the birth of Gabriela Valenzuela's baby?

- Click on **Return to Nurses' Station**.
- Click on **Chart** and then on **203** to view Kelly Brady's chart.
- Click on the **Physician's Notes** tab and review the note for Wednesday 1530.

Read the Cesarean Birth section on pages 181-183 in your textbook.

5. Why does Kelly Brady's physician now recommend immediate delivery?

6. What general risks related to cesarean section does Kelly Brady's physician discuss with her?

7. Because of Kelly Brady's early gestational age (26 weeks), her physician anticipates a classical uterine incision. How will this type of incision affect Kelly Brady's birth options in future pregnancies?

- Click on the **Physician's Orders** tab and review the orders for Wednesday 1540.

8. List the orders to be carried out before Kelly Brady's surgery. State the purpose of each order.

Order	Purpose

9. Can you think of other common preoperative procedures? List them below. (*Hint:* Refer to a basic medical-surgical textbook for ideas if you need help!)

Sexually Transmitted and Other Infections

Reading Assignment: Nursing Care of Women with Complications During Pregnancy (Chapter 5)
The Nurse's Role in Women's Health Care (Chapter 11)

Patients: Stacey Crider, Obstetrics Floor, Room 202
Gabriela Valenzuela, Obstetrics Floor, Room 205
Laura Wilson, Obstetrics Floor, Room 206

Objectives:

1. Assess and plan care for a pregnant woman with bacterial vaginosis.
2. Explain the importance of prophylactic group B streptococcus treatment.
3. Identify risk factors for acquiring HIV infection.
4. Prioritize information to be included in patient teaching related to HIV infection.

In this lesson, you will assess and evaluate the care provided to three hospitalized pregnant women, each of whom has a sexually transmitted infection (STI) or other vaginal infection.

Exercise 1

Virtual Hospital Activity

30 minutes

- Sign in to work at Pacific View Regional Hospital on the Obstetrics Floor for Period of Care 1. (*Note:* If you are already in the virtual hospital from a previous exercise, click on **Leave the Floor** and then on **Restart the Program** to get to the sign-in window.)
- From the Patient List, select Stacey Crider (Room 202).
- Click on **Go to Nurses' Station**.
- Click on **Chart** and then on **202** to view Stacey Crider's chart.
- Click on the **History and Physical** tab and review the information given.

1. In the table below, describe Stacey Crider's vaginal discharge on admission. How does it compare with the description of bacterial vaginosis (BV) found in Table 11-1 in your textbook?

	Stacey Crider's Discharge	**Textbook Description**
Appearance		
Amount		
Odor		

2. When discussing bacterial vaginosis with Stacey Crider, which statement by her would indicate an understanding of the condition?
   a. "This is a 'sex' disease much like gonorrhea or chlamydia."
   b. "I could get this from too much douching."
   c. "There is no cure for this infection."
   d. "Douching can help to manage my infection."

3. How is bacterial vaginosis diagnosed?

4. What medication is recommended for treating bacterial vaginosis during pregnancy?
   a. Metronidazole (Flagyl)
   b. Amoxicillin
   c. Cleocin
   d. Macrodantin

• Click on the **Physician's Orders** tab and review the admitting physician's orders on Tuesday at 0630.

5. What are Stacey Crider's admission diagnoses?

6. Explain how Stacey Crider's admission diagnoses are likely interrelated.

7. Which medication did Stacey Crider's physician order to treat her bacterial vaginosis?

- Click on **Return to Nurses' Station**.
- Click on the **Drug** icon in the lower left-hand corner of your screen and use the search box or scroll feature to locate the record for metronidazole.

8. _____ Treatment of Stacey Crider's sexual partner for bacterial vaginosis is not recommended. (True or False)

9. Assume that Stacey Crider is discharged home on day 4 of the prescribed treatment with this medication. What specific information about this drug should she be taught?

10. Common side effects associated with metronidazole therapy include which of the following?
    a. Diarrhea
    b. Vulvular swelling
    c. Metallic taste in the mouth
    d. Dry skin

Exercise 2

Virtual Hospital Activity

20 minutes

- Sign in to work at Pacific View Regional Hospital on the Obstetrics Floor for Period of Care 1. (*Note:* If you are already in the virtual hospital from a previous exercise, click on **Leave the Floor** and then on **Restart the Program** to get to the sign-in window.)
- From the Patient List, select Gabriela Valenzuela (Room 205).
- Click on **Go to Nurses' Station**.
- Click on **Chart** and then on **205** to view Gabriela Valenzuela's chart.
- Click on the **History and Physical** tab and review the plan outlined at the end of the document.

1. What is the medical plan of care for Gabriela Valenzuela?

2. Is Gabriela Valenzuela known to be positive for group B streptococcus (GBS)?

Read about group B streptococcus in your textbook.

3. List the risk factors for neonatal GBS infection.

4. Where can GBS be found in women? Select all that apply.

_____ Rectum

_____ Stomach

_____ Saliva

_____ Vagina

_____ Cervix

5. At what point in gestation is the pregnant woman cultured for the presence of GBS infection?
   a. During the first trimester
   b. 20-24 weeks gestation
   c. 24-28 weeks gestation
   d. 35-37 weeks gestation

6. Since pregnant women with GBS in the vagina are almost always asymptomatic, why does Gabriela Valenzuela need to be treated for this organism?

- Click on the **Physician's Orders** tab and review the admission orders for Tuesday at 2100.

7. What medication/dosage/frequency will Gabriela Valenzuela receive for Group B strep prophylaxis?

8. How does this order compare with the treatment regimen recommended in your textbook?

Exercise 3

Virtual Hospital Activity

20 minutes

- Sign in to work at Pacific View Regional Hospital on the Obstetrics Floor for Period of Care 1. (*Note:* If you are already in the virtual hospital from a previous exercise, click on **Leave the Floor** and then on **Restart the Program** to get to the sign-in window.)
- From the Patient List, select Laura Wilson (Room 206).
- Click on **Go to Nurses' Station**.
- Click on **Chart** and then on **206** to view Laura Wilson's chart.
- Click on the **Nursing Admission** tab and review the information given.

1. What risk factors for acquiring an STI are identified on Laura Wilson's Nursing Admission form?

2. List specific risk factors for acquiring HIV. Put an asterisk next to the risk factors that are present in Laura Wilson's history.

3. What did the admitting nurse document about Laura Wilson's knowledge and acceptance of her HIV diagnosis?

- Click on **Return to Nurses' Station**.
- Click on **206** at the bottom of the screen.
- Click on **Patient Care** and then on **Nurse-Client Interactions**.
- Select and view the video titled **0800: Teaching—HIV in Pregnancy**. (*Note:* Check the virtual clock to see whether enough time has elapsed. You can use the fast-forward feature to advance the time by 2-minute intervals if the video is not yet available. Then click again on **Patient Care** and **Nurse-Client Interactions** to refresh the screen.)

4. Does Laura Wilson appear to be fully aware of the implications of her HIV infection? State the rationale for your answer.

5. What coping mechanism is Laura Wilson exhibiting in the video?

- Click on **Chart** and then on **206** to view Laura Wilson's chart.
- Click on the **Nursing Admission** tab and review the information given.

6. Laura Wilson needs education on all of the listed topics. Which would you choose to teach her about at this time?
   a. Safer sex
   b. Medication side effects and importance of compliance
   c. Need for medical follow-up and medication for the baby
   d. Impact of HIV on birth plans

7. Give the rationale for your answer to the previous question.

Common Reproductive Concerns, Infertility, and Contraception

Reading Assignment: Human Reproductive Anatomy and Physiology (Chapter 2)
The Nurse's Role in Women's Health Care (Chapter 11)

Patients: Dorothy Grant, Obstetrics Floor, Room 201
Stacey Crider, Obstetrics Floor, Room 202
Kelly Brady, Obstetrics Floor, Room 203
Maggie Gardner, Obstetrics Floor, Room 204
Gabriela Valenzuela, Obstetrics Floor, Room 205
Laura Wilson, Obstetrics Floor, Room 206

Objectives:

1. Identify various reproductive concerns.

2. Differentiate among the various types of contraception that are available.

3. Identify various methods of testing and treatment options that can be used for couples experiencing infertility concerns.

Exercise 1

Virtual Hospital Activity

10 minutes

1. What causes the onset of menstruation?
   a. Increases in progesterone levels
   b. Decreases in progesterone levels
   c. Increases in estrogen levels
   d. Increases in luteinizing hormone levels

2. What is the average age for menarche?
   a. 10-14 years
   b. 11-15 years
   c. 12-15 years
   d. 13-16 years

3. The average menstrual cycle is _____ days.

4. What are the criteria for a diagnosis of amenorrhea?

- Sign in to work at Pacific View Regional Hospital on the Obstetrics Floor for Period of Care 1. (*Note:* If you are already in the virtual hospital from a previous exercise, click on **Leave the Floor** and then on **Restart the Program** to get to the sign-in window.)
- From the Patient List, select Stacey Crider (Room 202).
- Click on **Go to Nurses' Station**.
- Click on **Chart** and then on **202** to view Stacey Crider's chart.
- Click on the **History and Physical** tab and review the GYN History.

5. Does Stacey Crider meet the textbook criteria for amenorrhea?

6. What is her history?

Exercise 2

Virtual Hospital Activity

30 minutes

1. What is contraception?

- Sign in to work at Pacific View Regional Hospital on the Obstetrics Floor for Period of Care 1. (*Note:* If you are already in the virtual hospital from a previous exercise, click on **Leave the Floor** and then on **Restart the Program** to get to the sign-in window.)
- From the Patient List, select all six patients (although you will simply be reviewing the charts.)
- Click on **Go to Nurses' Station**.
- Click on **Chart** and then on **201** to view Dorothy Grant's chart.

- Click on the **History and Physical** tab and review the information on contraception.
- Repeat the previous three steps with each of the other five patients on the floor.

2. Below, list the birth control method each patient was using before this pregnancy.

Dorothy Grant

Stacey Crider

Kelly Brady

Maggie Gardner

Gabriela Valenzuela

Laura Wilson

3. What methods of contraception also provide protection against sexually transmitted infections (STIs)?

4. _____ is the only 100% effective method of preventing pregnancy and STIs.

5. Gabriela Valenzuela is a devout Catholic. Which method of birth control would be appropriate for the nurse to discuss with her?

6. When providing education concerning natural family planning, which should be included? Select all that apply.

_____ Natural family planning has a 30% failure rate.

_____ Most sperm will live 48 hours after ejaculation.

_____ Abstinence or barrier methods of contraception must be used during periods of high fertility.

_____ Basal body temperature will increase at ovulation and remain elevated for the last half of the cycle.

_____ Cervical mucus increases at ovulation.

7. Kelly Brady wants to use oral contraceptives to prevent pregnancy while she is breastfeeding. Which type of oral contraception is appropriate for her to use? Why?

8. Laura Wilson is HIV-positive. What is the most appropriate form of birth control for her? Why?

Exercise 3

Virtual Hospital Activity

45 minutes

1. Infertility is defined as the inability to conceive after what period of regular, unprotected sexual intercourse?
   a. 6 months
   b. 9 months
   c. 12 months
   d. 18 months

2. What are some psychological reactions to infertility?

3. List four factors that affect female fertility.

4. List four factors that affect male fertility.

- Sign in to work at Pacific View Regional Hospital on the Obstetrics Floor for Period of Care 1. (*Note:* If you are already in the virtual hospital from a previous exercise, click on **Leave the Floor** and then on **Restart the Program** to get to the sign-in window.)
- From the Patient List, select Maggie Gardner (Room 204).
- Click on **Go to Nurses' Station**.
- Click on **Chart** and then on **204** to view Maggie Gardner's chart.
- Click on the **History and Physical** tab and review the information given.

5. Maggie Gardner was married _____ years before conceiving the first time.

6. Based on the textbook reading, which would Maggie Gardner have been diagnosed with if she had chosen to get treatment after a year of attempting to get pregnant?
   a. Primary infertility
   b. Secondary infertility

7. List four factors that influence fertility.

8. Which of the above factors are known concerns with Maggie Gardner?

9. List at least four tests that can be completed on females to determine the causes of infertility.

10. List at least two tests that can be completed on males to determine the causes of infertility.

11. What test is used to assess couples to determine the adequacy of coital technique?

12. When is this test done?

13. What methods are available to assist the infertile couple in having a child?

14. What methods did Maggie Gardner and her husband use to assist them in getting pregnant? (*Hint:* Review the OB history in her History and Physical.)

Medication Administration

Reading Assignment: Nursing Care of Women with Complications During Pregnancy
(Chapter 5)

Patients: Dorothy Grant, Obstetrics Floor, Room 201
Stacey Crider, Obstetrics Floor, Room 202
Maggie Gardner, Obstetrics Floor, Room 204
Laura Wilson, Obstetrics Floor, Room 206

Objective:

1. Correctly administer selected medications to obstetric patients observing the six rights.

Exercise 1

Virtual Hospital Activity

30 minutes

- Sign in to work at Pacific View Regional Hospital on the Obstetrics Floor for Period of Care 2. (*Note:* If you are already in the virtual hospital from a previous exercise, click on **Leave the Floor** and then on **Restart the Program** to get to the sign-in window.)
- From the Patient List, select Dorothy Grant (Room 201).

Dorothy Grant was admitted at 30 weeks gestation for observation following blunt abdominal trauma (she was kicked in the abdomen by her husband). She is bleeding vaginally and may have sustained a placental abruption. Your assignment is to give Rhogam to Dorothy Grant. Read about Rhogam in your textbook. Use the Drug Guide as needed.

1. Rhogam is best classified as which category?
   a. Vaccine
   b. Antibiotic
   c. Immunoglobulin
   d. Corticosteroid

2. Which are indications for the administration of Rhogam? Select all that apply.

_____ An Rh-negative woman who has delivered an Rh-negative infant

_____ An Rh-negative woman who is 28 weeks gestation who has not experienced complications of pregnancy

_____ An Rh-positive woman whose history reflects a history of a blood transfusion within the past 2 years

_____ A woman who is Rh-negative and experienced sensitization during her last pregnancy

_____ An Rh-negative woman who has just had an amniocentesis

_____ An Rh-positive woman who has given birth to an Rh-negative infant

_____ An Rh-negative woman who has given birth to an Rh-positive infant

3. All of the following are scenarios in which Rh immune globulin might be administered. Which of these scenarios applies to Dorothy Grant?
   a. Administered within 72 hours of giving birth to an Rh-positive infant
   b. Given prophylactically at 28 weeks gestation
   c. Administered following an incident or exposure risk that occurs after 28 weeks gestation
   d. Given during first-trimester pregnancy following miscarriage, elective abortion, or ectopic pregnancy

4. What information must be confirmed about Dorothy Grant before giving her Rh immune globulin? Select all that apply.

_____ Rh status

_____ Number of past pregnancies

_____ Weight of newborn

_____ Antibody (Coombs) status

_____ Age

- Click on **Go to Nurses' Station**.
- Click on **Chart** and then on **201** to view Dorothy Grant's chart.
- Click on the **Physician's Orders** tab and review the orders for Wednesday 0730.

5. Write the physician's order for Rh immune globulin.

- Click on **Return to Nurses' Station**.
- Click on the **Drug** icon in the lower left-hand corner of your screen. Find the entry for Rh immune globulin and compare the physician's order for Dorothy Grant with the dosage and route specified in the Drug Guide.

6. According to the Drug Guide, does the physician's order use the correct dosage and route?

- Click on **Go to Nurses' Station** at the bottom of the screen.
- Click on **Chart** and then on **201** to view Dorothy Grant's chart.
- Click on the **Laboratory Reports** tab and review test results for 0245 Wednesday.

7. Dorothy Grant's blood type is _____.

8. What additional information do you need? Why? Is that information available?

- Click on **Return to Nurses' Station** and then on **Medication Room** at the bottom of your screen.
- Click on **Refrigerator** and open the refrigerator door.
- Click on **Put Medication on Tray** and then on **Close Door**.
- Click on **View Medication Room** and then on **Preparation**.
- Click on **Prepare** next to Rho(D) Immune Globulin and follow the prompts to complete preparation of this medication.
- Click on **Return to Medication Room** and then on **201** at the bottom of the screen to enter the patient's room.
- Click on **Check Armband**.
- Click on **Patient Care** and then on **Medication Administration**.

You are almost ready to give Dorothy Grant's injection. However, before you do . . .

9. _____ Rh immune globulin is often considered a blood product. (True or False)

- Find Rho(D) immune globulin in the list of medications set aside for Dorothy Grant.
- Click on the arrow next to Select and choose **Administer**.
- Follow the prompts to administer Dorothy Grant's injection. Check **Yes** to document this administration in the MAR.
- Click on **Leave the Floor** and then on **Look at Your Preceptor's Evaluation**.
- Click on **Medication Scorecard**. How did you do?
- Click on **Return to Evaluations** and then on **Return to Menu**.

Exercise 2

Virtual Hospital Activity

15 minutes

- Sign in to work at Pacific View Regional Hospital on the Obstetrics Floor for Period of Care 1. (*Note:* If you are already in the virtual hospital from a previous exercise, click on **Leave the Floor** and then on **Restart the Program** to get to the sign-in window.)
- From the Patient List, select Maggie Gardner (Room 204).
- Click on **Go to Nurses' Station**.
- Click on **Chart** and then on **204** to view Maggie Gardner's chart.
- Click on the **Nursing Admission** tab and review the information given.

1. Maggie Gardner repeatedly expresses anxiety throughout the Nursing Admission. What is her primary concern? Why? Provide documentation.

2. Maggie Gardner states that before this pregnancy she had a highly adaptive coping mechanism. How does she rate her ability to cope at this point? Why? (*Hint:* See the Coping and Stress Tolerance section in the Nursing Admission.)

- Click on the **Physician's Orders** tab and review the information given.

3. What medication has the physician ordered to help Maggie Gardner with her anxiety?

- Click on **Return to Nurses' Station**.
- Click on the **Drug** icon in the lower left corner of your screen.
- Use the search box or the scroll bar to find the medication you identified in the previous question.

4. What is the drug's mechanism of action?

- Click on **Return to Nurses' Station** and then on **204** at the bottom of the screen to enter Maggie Gardner's room.
- Click on **Patient Care** and then on **Nurse-Client Interactions**.

- Select and view the video titled **0745: Evaluation—Efficacy of Drugs**. (*Note:* Check the virtual clock to see whether enough time has elapsed. You can use the fast-forward feature to advance the time by 2-minute intervals if the video is not yet available. Then click again on **Patient Care** and **Nurse-Client Interactions** to refresh the screen.)

5. According to the nurse, how long will it take for Maggie Gardner to see therapeutic effects of the drug? How does this correlate with what you learned in the Teaching section of the Drug Guide?

Exercise 3

Virtual Hospital Activity

20 minutes

- Sign in to work at Pacific View Regional Hospital on the Obstetrics Floor for Period of Care 1. (*Note:* If you are already in the virtual hospital from a previous exercise, click on **Leave the Floor** and then on **Restart the Program** to get to the sign-in window.)
- From the Patient List, select Stacey Crider (Room 202).

1. In this exercise, you will administer betamethasone to Stacey Crider, who was admitted to the hospital at 27 weeks gestation in preterm labor. Before preparing Stacey Crider's betamethasone, what do you need to do?

- Click on **Go to Nurses' Station**.
- Click on **Chart** and then on **202** to view Stacey Crider's chart.
- Click on the **Physician's Orders** tab and find the order for betamethasone.

2. After verifying the Physician's Order, what is your next step?

- Click on **Return to Nurses' Station** and then on **Medication Room** at the bottom of your screen.
- Click on **Unit Dosage** and then on drawer **202**.
- Select **Betamethasone**; then click on **Put Medication on Tray**.
- Click on **Close Drawer**.
- Click on **View Medication Room** and then on **Preparation**.
- Click on **Prepare** and follow the prompts to complete preparation of Stacey Crider's betamethasone dose.
- Click on **Return to Medication Room**.

3. Now that the medication is prepared, what is your next step?

- Click on **202** to enter the patient's room.
- Click on **Check Armband** and then on **Check Allergies**.
- Click on **Patient Care** and then on **Medication Administration**.
- Click **Select** for betamethasone and choose **Administer**.

4. What's the final step in the process?

- If you haven't already, indicate **Yes** to document this administration in the MAR.
- Click on **Leave the Floor**.
- Click on **Look at Your Preceptor's Evaluation**.
- Click on **Medication Scorecard**. How did you do?
- Click on **Return to Evaluations** and then on **Return to Menu.**

Exercise 4

Virtual Hospital Activity

30 minutes

- Sign in to work at Pacific View Regional Hospital on the Obstetrics Floor for Period of Care 1. (*Note:* If you are already in the virtual hospital from a previous exercise, click on **Leave the Floor** and then on **Restart the Program** to get to the sign-in window.)
- From the Patient List, select Laura Wilson (Room 206).
- Click on **Go to Nurses' Station**.
- Click on **MAR** and then on **206** to view Laura Wilson's MAR.

1. Laura Wilson's medications for Wednesday include several different types of drugs. Which of the following is used to treat her HIV-positive status?
   a. Zidovudine 200 mg PO every 8 hours
   b. Prenatal multivitamin 1 tablet PO daily
   c. Lactated Ringer's 75 mL/hr IV continuous

- Click on **Return to Nurses' Station**.
- Click on the **Drug** icon in the lower left corner of the screen.
- Use the search box or scroll bar to find the medication you identified in the previous question.

2. What is the drug's mechanism of action?

3. What is the drug's therapeutic effect?

4. Does this medication cross the placenta? Is it distributed in breast milk?

5. What symptoms/side effects of this medication need to be reported to the physician?

6. How should this medication be taken?

7. Your final assignment is to give Laura Wilson the medication that is due at 0800. During these lessons, we have provided you with detailed instructions on how to give medications. Now it is time for you to fly solo. Don't forget the six rights of medication administration . . . and have fun! Document below how you did.

Note: If you'd like to get more practice, there are other medications that can be given at the beginning of the first three periods of care. Below is a list of the patients, medications, routes of administration, and administration times that can be used. As you practice, be sure to select the correct patient when you sign in. That way, you can get a Medication Scorecard for evaluation after you prepare and administer a medication. (*Remember:* If you need help at any time, refer to the **Getting Started** section of this workbook.)

PERIOD OF CARE 1

Dorothy Grant (Room 201)

- Betamethasone 12 mg IM
- Prenatal multivitamin PO

Stacey Crider (Room 202)

- 0800: Prenatal multivitamin PO
- Metronidazole 500 mg PO
- Betamethasone 12 mg IM
- Insulin lispro subQ
- Nifedipine 20 mg PO

Kelly Brady (Room 203)

- 0730/0800: Prenatal multivitamin PO
- Ferrous sulfate PO
- Labetalol hydrochloride 400 mg PO
- Nifedipine 10 mg PO

Maggie Gardner (Room 204)

- 0800: Prenatal multivitamin PO
- Buspirone hydrochloride 7.5 mg PO

Gabriela Valenzuela (Room 205)

- 0800: Ampicillin 2 grams IV
- Betamethasone 12 mg IM
- Prenatal multivitamin PO

Laura Wilson (Room 206)

- Zidovudine 200 mg PO
- Prenatal multivitamin PO

PERIOD OF CARE 2

Dorothy Grant (Room 201)

- 1200: Rho(D) immune globulin IM

Stacey Crider (Room 202)

- 1200: Insulin lispro subQ

Kelly Brady (Room 203)

- 1130: Betamethasone 12 mg IM

Maggie Gardner (Room 204)

- 1115: Prednisone 40 mg PO
- Aspirin 81 mg PO

PERIOD OF CARE 3

Maggie Gardner (Room 204)

- 1500: Buspirone 7.5 mg PO

LESSON 12

Caring for an Infant with Bronchiolitis

Reading Assignment: An Overview of Growth, Development, and Nutrition (Chapter 15)
The Infant (Chapter 16)
Health Care Adaptations for the Child and Family (Chapter 22)
The Child with a Respiratory Disorder (Chapter 25)
Childhood Communicable Diseases, Bioterrorism, Natural Disasters, and the Maternal-Child Patient (Chapter 32)

Patient: Carrie Richards, Pediatrics Floor, Room 303

Objectives:

1. Discuss the pathophysiology of bronchiolitis.
2. Explain the role of respiratory syncytial virus (RSV) in bronchiolitis.
3. Relate the effect of an infant's level of growth and development on bronchiolitis.
4. Complete a respiratory assessment on an infant and discuss nursing care issues.
5. Determine nursing interventions for an infant with bronchiolitis.

In this lesson you will learn and reinforce concepts related to a common respiratory illness in infants. You will apply principles of growth and development in making nursing care decisions. You will be expected to recall/review basic oral and written communication skills, teaching skills, and family-centered care. Your patient is Carrie Richards, a 3½-month-old who has been admitted to the Pediatric Unit from the Emergency Department. Carrie Richards' medical diagnosis is bronchiolitis. Her mother is with her.

Exercise 1

Writing Activity

10 minutes

1. Explain the pathophysiology of bronchiolitis.

2. What is the relationship between respiratory syncytial virus (RSV) and bronchiolitis?

3. Discuss infant growth and development as it relates to respiratory tract function.

Exercise 2

Virtual Hospital Activity

20 minutes

- Sign in to work at Pacific View Regional Hospital on the Pediatrics Floor for Period of Care 1. (*Note:* If you are already in the virtual hospital from a previous exercise, click on **Leave the Floor** and then on **Restart the Program** to get to the sign-in window.)
- From the Patient List, select Carrie Richards (Room 303).
- Click on **Go to Nurses' Station**.
- Click on **Chart** and then on **303**.
- Click on the **Emergency Department** tab and review the record.
- Click on and review the **Physician's Orders**, **History and Physical**, and **Nursing Admission**.

1. As you review these records, list the data that are consistent with bronchiolitis.

2. What do these observations indicate as far as Carrie Richards' health status is concerned? Do you think Carrie Richards is mildly or severely ill? Explain.

- Click on the **Physician's Orders** and find the medications ordered for Carrie Richards.
- Click on **Return to Nurses' Station**.
- Click on the **Drug** icon in the lower left corner of your screen to review the ordered medications. (*Hint:* You may also refer to a nursing drug handbook if you need more information.)

3. What are the rationales for the orders for IV fluid, medications, pulse oximetry, and lab work?

4. Nasal washing was performed on Carrie Richards while she was in the Emergency Department. If you were assisting with the nasal washing procedure, would you anticipate restraining her? If so, how? Would you have Carrie Richards' mother help? What factors would you consider in deciding what to do? (*Hint:* Check Carrie Richards' physical status and behavior while she was in the Emergency Department.)

5. Which is consistent with the type of isolation being used for Carrie Richards? Select all that apply. (*Hint:* Review the Physician's Orders in her chart.)

_____   Private room only

_____   Semi-private room with another patient who has the same infection

_____   Use of clean gloves

_____   Use of sterile gloves

_____   Negative air flow room

_____   Wearing of a gown when anticipating contact with patient or contaminated surfaces

6. What other infection-control precautions, aside from isolation, need to be implemented?

7. What is a nosocomial infection, and why must care be taken to prevent Carrie Richards from developing one?

- Click on **Return to Nurses' Station** and then on **303** at the bottom of the screen.
- Click on **Patient Care** and then on **Nurse-Client Interactions**.
- Select and view the video titled **0730: Patient Assessment**. (*Note:* Check the virtual clock to see whether enough time has elapsed. You can use the fast-forward feature to advance the time by 2-minute intervals if the video is not yet available. Then click again on **Patient Care** and **Nurse-Client Interactions** to refresh the screen.)

8. In this video, what are the nurse and Carrie Richards' mother doing right? What are they doing wrong?

Exercise 3

Virtual Hospital Activity

45 minutes

- Sign in to work at Pacific View Regional Hospital on the Pediatrics Floor for Period of Care 1. (*Note:* If you are already in the virtual hospital from a previous exercise, click on **Leave the Floor** and then on **Restart the Program** to get to the sign-in window.)
- From the Patient List, select Carrie Richards (Room 303).
- Click on **Go to Nurses' Station**.
- Click on **303** to go to Carrie Richards' room.
- Inside the room, click on **Check Armband** and then on **Take Vital Signs**. Note Carrie Richards' vital signs for documentation.
- Next, click on **Patient Care** and perform a head-to-toe assessment by clicking on the various body system categories (yellow buttons) and body system subcategories (green buttons).

1. Based on your assessment, list any observations that reflect the status of Carrie Richards' oxygenation.

2. When performing the assessment on Carrie Richards, which of the following developmental findings are normal for her age? Select all that apply.

_____ Reaches for overhead objects with fingers

_____ Prefers to look at familiar sights

_____ Holds hands open most of the time

_____ Elevates self with arms

_____ Sits alone momentarily

3. When taking Carrie Richards' temperature, which method is the most appropriate to use?
   a. Axillary
   b. Oral
   c. Rectal
   d. Tympanic

4. What is the proper position to hold the pinna of the ear when using a tympanic thermometer on Carrie Richards?
   a. Down and back
   b. Up and back
   c. Straight back

5. What are Carrie Richards' vital signs? Are they within normal range for her age?

6. Carrie Richards is of African-American descent. What is the best way to assess color in a dark-skinned person?

- Click on **EPR** and then on **Login**.
- Specify **303** from the Patient drop-down menu.
- Begin charting the findings from your assessment of Carrie Richards by selecting **Vital Signs** from the Category drop-down menu. Use the blue backward and forward arrows as needed to document these data in the appropriate time columns.
- Continue to chart your observations in the Respiratory and Cardiovascular categories.

7. If you missed anything, go back to Carrie Richards' room and reassess her. Because the EPR format is generic, you may not have data for all areas listed. Even so, you do need to make sure you are recognizing significant assessment data. Review data trends since admission. Why is continued monitoring necessary?

- Click on **Exit EPR** to return to Carrie Richards' room.
- Based on your previous findings and your answer to question 7, perform a focused assessment of Carrie Richards.
- Click on **Leave the Floor**.
- Click on **Look at Your Preceptor's Evaluation**s.
- Click on and review the **Examination Report**.

8. How did you do with your focused assessment? Do you note any gaps? Were you efficient and systemic? Is there any need for improvement in your performance? If so, in what areas?

- Click on **Return to Evaluations**.
- Click on **Return to Menu** and then on **Restart the Program**.
- Sign in to work at Pacific View Regional Hospital on the Pediatric Floor for Period of Care 1.
- From the Patient List, select Carrie Richards (Room 303).
- Click on **Go to Nurses' Station**.
- Click on **EPR** and then on **Login**.
- Select **303** from the Patient drop-down menu and document your latest assessment findings.

9. In the event that Carrie Richards' condition begins to deteriorate, what changes might be anticipated? Select all that apply.

_____ Decrease in heart rate

_____ Nasal flaring

_____ Increasing respiratory rate with activity

_____ Decrease in pulse oximetry reading

_____ Restlessness

_____ Cyanosis of nailbeds

10. _____ Carrie Richards' condition can be described as deteriorating. (True or False)

11. Carrie Richards is at risk for dehydration. What parameters must be included in the observation of the condition?

12. How is Carrie Richards receiving oxygen?

13. Sometimes oxygen is delivered using a mist tent. What are the nursing responsibilities for care of an infant in a mist tent? Are there any advantages to using a mist tent rather than a nasal cannula?

14. How is Carrie Richards' O_2 status being monitored? What should the nurse be looking for?

15. Documentation is important. What information is necessary for documenting observations associated with Carrie Richards' O_2 saturation levels?

16. Oxygenation assessment is ongoing. In older children and adults, the nurse can easily assess respiratory status in response to play or other activity. How can this ongoing assessment be carried out in an infant?

17. Develop a list of the major nursing interventions for Carrie Richards.

Nursing Care Issues Associated with Bronchiolitis

Reading Assignment: An Overview of Growth, Development, and Nutrition (Chapter 15)
The Infant (Chapter 16)
Health Care Adaptations for the Child and Family (Chapter 22)
The Child with a Respiratory Disorder (Chapter 25)
Childhood Communicable Diseases, Bioterrorism, Natural Disasters, and
the Maternal-Child Patient (Chapter 32)

Patient: Carrie Richards, Pediatrics Floor, Room 303

Objectives:

1. Discuss the reasons why infants are at risk for hydration problems.
2. Explain the risk for dehydration in infants with respiratory problems.
3. Discuss nursing care for managing hydration concerns, including IV therapy.
4. Practice oral medication administration in infants.
5. Identify and discuss teaching implications in the care of infants.
6. Discuss discharge information for the parent(s) of a patient with bronchiolitis.

In this lesson you will explore hydration as an area of concern for infants with respiratory problems. You will also explore oral medication administration and practice it in the virtual hospital setting. You will consider the role of the nurse related to a variety of teaching areas: the illness, oral administration of medications, and growth and development. You will need to recall and use the principles of good communication and family teaching as you continue to work with Carrie Richards.

Exercise 1

Writing Activity

20 minutes

1. Which characteristics of infants put them at a greater risk for hydration problems? Select all that apply.

   _____ Infants have a larger body surface area, which results in greater fluid loss through the skin.

   _____ The metabolic rate of an infant is lower than that of an adult.

   _____ Infants have a higher percentage of water in extracellular fluid.

   _____ Infants are less able to concentrate urine.

2. Which is the most reliable information that can be used to assess an infant's hydration over time?
   a. Weight of wet diapers
   b. Daily weight
   c. Urine osmolality readings
   d. Assessment of oral mucous membranes

3. When weighing an infant, what practices will promote the most accurate readings? Select all that apply.

   _____ Weigh at the same time each day

   _____ Weigh after feedings

   _____ Weigh with the infant in a diaper only

   _____ Weigh the infant without clothing or diaper

4. Explain what is meant by oral rehydration therapy (ORT).

5. Discuss the nursing responsibilities associated with IV fluid administration in infants. (*Hint:* Remember that IV fluid is treated as a medication administration.)

6. What should the nurse be looking for when assessing an IV site?

7. What topics should be included in the discharge instructions for the parents of an infant who has been hospitalized with bronchiolitis?

Exercise 2

Virtual Hospital Activity

30 minutes

- Sign in to work at Pacific View Regional Hospital on the Pediatrics Floor for Period of Care 1. (*Note:* If you are already in the virtual hospital from a previous exercise, click on **Leave the Floor** and then on **Restart the Program** to get to the sign-in window.)
- From the Patient List, select Carrie Richards (Room 303).
- Click on **Get Report** and review the Clinical Report.
- Click on **Go to Nurses' Station**.
- Click on **303** at the bottom of your screen.
- Click on **Patient Care** and complete a focused assessment of Carrie Richards by clicking on the various body system categories (yellow buttons) and then on the body system subcategories (green buttons). (*Remember:* A focused assessment is one that reflects the priority health concern as well as those concerns for which the patient is at risk.)

- Once your assessment is complete, click on **EPR** and then on **Login**.
- Select Carrie Richards' room number (**303**) from the Patient drop-down menu and choose categories as needed from the Category drop-down menu to record the data from your focused assessment. (*Hint:* If you need help entering data in the EPR, refer to pages 15-16 in the **Getting Started** section of this workbook.)
- When you have finished documenting your assessments, click on **Exit EPR**.
- Now, to see how you did, first click on **Leave the Floor**.
- From the Floor Menu, select **Look at Your Preceptor's Evaluation**s.
- Click on **Examination Report** and review the feedback.

1. Reflect on your performance with this assessment. Did you assess respiratory status along with hydration parameters? Remember that each affects the other.

2. What important hydration assessment parameters can you use with Carrie Richards that would not be available with an older child?

Now let's jump ahead in virtual time to practice your focused assessment again.

- Click on **Return to Evaluations**, **Return to Menu**, and then **Restart the Program**.
- Sign in to work on the Pediatrics Floor for Period of Care 2.
- From the Patient List, select Carrie Richards (Room 303).
- Click on **Go to Nurses' Station** and then on **303** at the bottom of the screen to enter Carrie Richards' room.
- Click on **Patient Care** and complete a focused assessment. Then chart your findings on the appropriate flow sheets in the EPR.
- When you have finished documenting your assessments, click on **Exit EPR**.
- Now, see how you did. Click on **Leave the Floor**.
- From the Floor Menu, select **Look at Your Preceptor's Evaluation**s.
- Click on **Examination Report** and review the feedback.

3. Reflect on how you are doing with your focused assessment. Consider completeness, comfort, efficiency, and skill. Are you feeling more confident about your thoroughness?

4. You know that infusion pumps are in very short supply. You also know that Carrie Richards, because of her age, needs a pump and will get the next one that becomes available. In the meantime, she has IV tubing with a burette. What is the rationale for use of this type of tubing?

5. When evaluating Carrie Richards' output, the nurse recognizes that she should have at least

   _____ wet diapers per day.

6. What would you tell Carrie Richards' mother about adequate hydration? How will she know whether or not her baby is getting enough fluids?

7. Carrie Richards is receiving an IV infusion with potassium added. Explain what she is receiving. Discuss the nurse's responsibilities related to potassium administration to an infant.

8. What can Carrie Richards' mother do regarding management of the IV? What could you ask her to do while still maintaining safe care and fulfilling your legal responsibility?

Exercise 3

Virtual Hospital Activity

45 minutes

- Sign in to work at Pacific View Regional Hospital on the Pediatrics Floor for Period of Care 3. (*Note:* If you are already in the virtual hospital from a previous exercise, click on **Leave the Floor** and then on **Restart the Program** to get to the sign-in window.)
- From the Patient List, select Carrie Richards (Room 303).
- Click on **Go to Nurses' Station**.
- Click on **303** to go to Carrie Richards' room.
- Click on **Take Vital Signs**.
- Click on **Clinical Alerts** and review the report.

1. Can Carrie Richards be given acetaminophen? If so, for what reason?

2. What should you assess before you prepare the medication? (*Hint:* Consider the specific need for this medication, as well as the nursing responsibilities before administering any medication.)

• Click on **MAR** and then on **303**. Find the order for this medication.

3. Is the ordered dose of this medication appropriate for Carrie Richards? Why or why not?

4. Assume that Carrie Richards has an order for an antibiotic that reads "40 mg/kg/day PO in divided doses every 8 hours." How much would you give for each dose?

5. What are the appropriate methods for administering oral medications to an infant?

- Click on **Return to Room 303**.
- Click on **Medication Room**.
- Click on **Unit Dosage** and then on drawer **303**.
- Select **Acetaminophen** and then click on **Put Medication on Tray**.
- Click on **Close Drawer**.
- Click on **View Medication Room**; then click **Preparation**.
- Click on **Prepare** and follow the Preparation Wizard's prompts.
- Click on **Return to Medication Room**.
- Click on **303** to return to Carrie Richards' room.
- Click on **Check Armband** and **Check Allergies**.
- Click on **Patient Care** and then on **Medication Administration**.
- Find Acetaminophen listed on the left side of your screen. Click on the down arrow next to Select and choose **Administer**.
- Follow the Administration Wizard's prompts to administer the medication. Indicate **Yes** to document this administration in the MAR.
- Click on **Leave the Floor**.
- Click on **Look at Your Preceptor's Evaluation**.
- Click on **Medication Scorecard**. How did you do?
- Click on **Return to Evaluations** and then on **Return to Menu**.

6. Did you get check marks indicating that you completed the medication administration procedure satisfactorily? What, if anything, did you forget? What, if anything, would you do differently?

You have just been walked through the medication preparation and administration procedure. Now try it on your own. You can practice preparing and giving Carrie Richards the same acetaminophen dose you just completed, or you can check the MAR to see whether there are any other medications that you can administer to her.

- Click on **Restart the Program**.
- Sign in to work on the Pediatrics Floor for Period of Care 3.
- From the Patient List, select Carrie Richards (Room 303) and proceed from there.
- Remember to follow the six rights! After you have finished administering the medication, be sure to see how you did by checking your Medication Scorecard.

Now let's jump backward in virtual time to visit Carrie Richards earlier in the day.

- Sign in to work at Pacific View Regional Hospital on the Pediatrics Floor for Period of Care 2.
- From the Patient List, select Carrie Richards (Room 303).
- Click on **Go to Nurses' Station** and then on **303** at the bottom of the screen to go to Carrie Richards's room.
- Click on **Patient Care** and then on **Nurse-Client Interactions**.
- Select and view the video titled **1115: Nutritional Assessment**. (*Note:* Check the virtual clock to see whether enough time has elapsed. You can use the fast-forward feature to advance the time by 2-minute intervals if the video is not yet available. Then click again on **Patient Care** and **Nurse-Client Interactions** to refresh the screen.)

7. Share your thoughts on the nurse's teaching. Consider the teaching-learning principles that are depicted.

8. Carrie Richards' mother needs to know how to give medication to her child at home. How will you determine whether she is skillful and comfortable enough giving her baby medication?

9. How would you respond to the following concern: "The nurse is supposed to give the medication, so how can the nurse allow a parent to administer medication?" (*Hint:* To answer this, you need to think through the nurse's legal responsibilities.)

10. The only vaccine Carrie Richards has received is for hepatitis B. What teaching does Carrie Richards' mother need with regard to immunizations?

11. What other kinds of information would you want from Carrie Richards' mother? (*Hint:* Explore other factors contributing to her behavior and decision making.)

12. Suppose that Carrie Richards' mother expresses concern about pain. She says that she avoids bringing her daughter in for shots because of this fear. You have shared this information, and the RN has requested an order for EMLA cream to be applied prior to any injections. What information does Carrie Richards' mother need in order to use EMLA cream?

Caring for an Infant Who Is Failing to Thrive

Reading Assignment: An Overview of Growth, Development, and Nutrition (Chapter 15)
The Child with a Gastrointestinal Condition (Chapter 28)

Patient: Carrie Richards, Pediatrics Floor, Room 303

Objectives:

1. Discuss the normal nutritional needs of the infant.
2. Define failure to thrive (FTT).
3. Consider patterns of growth that may indicate FTT.
4. Determine areas of assessment when FTT is suspected.
5. Discuss the relationship between parenting skills and FTT.
6. Develop specific interventions for caring for an infant with FTT.

As you complete this lesson, you will explore the complexities of failure to thrive, including the factors of parent-infant interaction and parenting skills. You will also consider the role of the nurse in assessment, support, and teaching when providing care.

Exercise 1

Writing Activity

30 minutes

1. Why is adequate nutrition especially important in infancy?

2. Describe appropriate nutritional intake for an infant at 3½ months of age.

3. Which statements concerning organic and nonorganic failure to thrive (FTT) are correct? Select all that apply.

_____ Organic FTT is characterized by failure to gain weight.

_____ Organic FTT is associated by a failure to gain weight secondary to physical factors such as cardiac disease or malabsorption.

_____ Non-organic FTT may be caused by parental neglect.

_____ Failure to thrive is seen with higher percentages in autistic children

_____ Children with certain personality types have failure to thrive issues

4. The following is a list of physiological and psychosocial assessment data. Place an X next to each piece of data that should be assessed further when there is a concern about failure to thrive. Select all that apply.

_____ Weight less than 3rd to 5th percentile

_____ Sudden deceleration in growth or weight loss

_____ Delay in reaching milestones

_____ Decreased muscle mass

_____ Muscle hypotonia

_____ Wary of caregivers

_____ Unresponsive to cuddling

_____ Nonnurturing parenting behaviors

_____ Avoidance of eye contact or touch

_____ Intense watchfulness

_____ Sleep disturbance

_____ Lack of age-appropriate stranger anxiety

_____ Lack of preference for parents

5. Are there other areas that need to be assessed? If so, list some of these areas.

6. _____ An inability to meet developmental tasks may result from FTT. (True or False)

7. What is the nurse's responsibility if there is a suspicion of abuse? (*Hint:* Discuss documentation and reporting.)

8. Discuss your own thoughts and any possible biases concerning child abuse and neglect.

Exercise 2

Virtual Hospital Activity

20 minutes

- Sign in to work at Pacific View Regional Hospital on the Pediatrics Floor for Period of Care 2. (*Note:* If you are already in the virtual hospital from a previous exercise, click on **Leave the Floor** and then on **Restart the Program** to get to the sign-in window.)
- From the Patient List, select Carrie Richards (Room 303).
- Click on **Go to Nurses' Station**.
- Click on **Chart** and then on **303**.
- Click on **Nursing Admission**.

1. If you knew Carrie Richards' birth weight, how would you use this information for assessment? What is the rule of thumb for expected weight gain in an infant during the first year of life?

2. Discuss the potential role of an interdisciplinary team providing care for Carrie Richards. Who might be involved?

- Now click on **Consultations**.
- Review the Dietary/Nutrition Consult.

3. Find Carrie Richards' birth weight and current weight. Based on this information, what concerns do you have about her rate of growth?

4. You considered the recommended diet for a 3½-month-old in question 2 of Exercise 1 in this lesson. How does this compare with Carrie Richards' diet? Evaluate the adequacy of her diet and consider her mother's rationales for these choices. Is there anything else you want to know or assess?

5. Based on your review of the Dietary/Nutrition Consult, what do you think is the problem in regard to Carrie Richards' feedings? What additional dietary recommendations are planned for her?

6. As you talk with Carrie Richards' mother, you learn that income is a problem. When discussing feeding, what should you incorporate in your teaching?

7. How will you teach Carrie Richards' mother about formula preparation?

Exercise 3

Virtual Hospital Activity

20 minutes

- Sign in to work at Pacific View Regional Hospital on the Pediatrics Floor for Period of Care 1. (*Note:* If you are already in the virtual hospital from a previous exercise, click on **Leave the Floor** and then on **Restart the Program** to get to the sign-in window.)
- From the Patient List, select Carrie Richards (Room 303).
- Click on **Go to Nurses' Station**.
- Click on **Chart** and then on **303**.
- Review the **History and Physical**.

1. Based on your review of the patient's chart and the FTT assessment data that you identified in the previous exercise, place an X next to any data that are consistent with FTT in Carrie Richards' case. Select all that apply.

_____ Weight less than 3rd to 5th percentile

_____ Sudden deceleration in growth or weight loss

_____ Delay in reaching milestones

_____ Decreased muscle mass

_____ Muscle hypotonia

_____ Wary of caregivers

_____ Unresponsive to cuddling

_____ Nonnurturing parenting behaviors

_____ Avoidance of eye contact or touch

_____ Intense watchfulness

_____ Sleep disturbance

_____ Lack of age-appropriate stranger anxiety

_____ Lack of preference for parents

- Click on **Return to Nurses' Station** and then on **303** at the bottom of the screen.
- Click on **Patient Care** and then on **Nurse-Client Interactions**.
- Select and view the video titled **0755: Intervention—Weight**. (*Note:* Check the virtual clock to see whether enough time has elapsed. You can use the fast-forward feature to advance the time by 2-minute intervals if the video is not yet available. Then click again on **Patient Care** and **Nurse-Client Interactions** to refresh the screen.)
- Now select and view the video titled **0800: Assessment—Fact Finding**. (*Note:* Check the virtual clock to see whether enough time has elapsed. You can use the fast-forward feature to advance the time by 2-minute intervals if the video is not yet available. Then click again on **Patient Care** and **Nurse-Client Interactions** to refresh the screen.)

2. What do you think the nurse is assessing as she observes the mother feeding Carrie Richards?

3. Why is it essential to know that Carrie Richards' mother is able to respond to her infant's cues and correctly interpret them?

4. A nursing care plan has been started for Carrie Richards. One nursing diagnosis is Ineffective coping related to decreased income and lack of support. The goals are for Carrie Richards' mother to identify resources and support systems available to her. What interventions would you anticipate finding in her care plan?

5. What if you noticed that Carrie Richards' mother always had the television on while feeding Carrie Richards and seemed to pay more attention to the TV than to her daughter? How would you intervene?

6. Envision yourself working with Carrie Richards' mother. How do you feel toward her? What do you think it would be like to carry out this nursing care? (*Hint:* Think about what the term "Rescue Fantasy" means to you.)

15

Caring for a Young Child with Meningitis

Reading Assignment: The Toddler (Chapter 17)
The Preschool Child (Chapter 18)
The Child's Experience of Hospitalization (Chapter 21)
Health Care Adaptations for the Child and Family (Chapter 22)
The Child with a Sensory or Neurological Condition (Chapter 23)

Patient: Stephanie Brown, Pediatrics Floor, Room 304

Objectives:

1. Describe the pathophysiology of meningitis.
2. Discuss risk factors for meningitis.
3. List assessment data indicative of meningitis.
4. Explain the rationale for treatment of meningitis.
5. Develop interventions for caring for a child with meningitis.
6. Discuss strategies for supporting a parent and child through diagnosis and treatment.

In this lesson you will learn about the problem of meningitis in a child and the related nursing care. You will focus on a variety of challenges associated with this problem. You may need to review the concepts of growth and development of a young child, as well as teaching-learning principles.

Exercise 1

Writing Activity

10 minutes

1. Review the pathophysiology of meningitis in your textbook. Which statements about meningitis are correct? Select all that apply.

    _____ Meningitis is an inflammation of the brain.

    _____ Bacterial meningitis is most common in teens.

    _____ Bacterial meningitis peaks in children from 6 to 12 months of age.

    _____ A dental infection can potentially lead to meningitis.

    _____ Staphylococcus is the leading cause of meningitis in children.

2. A series of tests have been ordered to confirm a diagnosis of meningitis. Which characteristic in the cerebral spinal fluid is consistent with the diagnosis of meningitis?
    a. Clear
    b. Increased protein levels
    c. Increased glucose levels
    d. Decreased cerebral spinal fluid pressure

3. Which signs and symptoms must the nurse recognize when caring for the patient with meningitis? Select all that apply.

    _____ Elevated temperature

    _____ Nuchal rigidity

    _____ Irritability

    _____ Hypotension

    _____ Petechiae

    _____ Drowsiness

Exercise 2

Virtual Hospital Activity

20 minutes

- Sign in to work at Pacific View Regional Hospital on the Pediatrics Floor for Period of Care 1. (*Note:* If you are already in the virtual hospital from a previous exercise, click on **Leave the Floor** and then on **Restart the Program** to get to the sign-in window.)
- From the Patient List, select Stephanie Brown (Room 304).
- Click on **Get Report** and review the information given.
- Click on **Go to Nurses' Station**.
- Click on **Chart** and then on **304**.
- Click on and review the following sections of the chart: **Physician's Notes**, **Emergency Department**, **History and Physical**, and **Nursing Admission**.

1. What assessment data did Stephanie Brown exhibit on admission that would indicate a diagnosis of meningitis?

2. Increased intracranial pressure (ICP) is a potential concern in a child with meningitis. What findings may be indicative of increased ICP? Select all that apply.

_____   Increased heart rate

_____   Decreased heart rate

_____   Increased respiratory rate

_____   Decreased respiratory rate

_____   Increased blood pressure

_____   Decreased blood pressure

3. If Stephanie Brown were an infant, what other assessments should you perform?

- Click on **Return to Nurses' Station** and then on **304** at the bottom of the screen.
- Click on **Take Vital Signs**.
- Review Stephanie Brown's vital signs.

4. Do any of Stephanie Brown's vital signs need to be reported immediately? Why or why not?

- Click on **Chart** and then on **304** to return to Stephanie Brown's chart.
- Click on the **Physician's Orders** tab and review the information given.
- Then click on the **Diagnostic Reports** tab and review the information there.

5. You are to assist the physician with a spinal lumbar puncture procedure. List your responsibilities.

6. How should you anticipate positioning and supporting Stephanie Brown through the lumbar puncture procedure?

7. Match each of the following physician's orders with its rationale.

Physician's Order	Rationale
_____ Pulse oximetry every 4 hours	a. Baseline (aminoglycosides can cause ototoxicity)
_____ Neuro checks every 4 hours	b. To reduce intracranial pressure
_____ Blood culture for fever above 101 degrees	c. To maintain therapeutic blood level
_____ Audiogram	d. Monitoring of neurological status
_____ HOB elevated 45 degrees	e. To prevent disease transmission via droplets
_____ Respiratory isolation	f. Assessment for other causative agents
_____ Vancomycin levels	g. Ongoing monitoring of O_2 status

Exercise 3

Virtual Hospital Activity

45 minutes

- Sign in to work at Pacific View Regional Hospital on the Pediatrics Floor for Period of Care 1. (*Note:* If you are already in the virtual hospital from a previous exercise, click on **Leave the Floor** and then on **Restart the Program** to get to the sign-in window.)
- From the Patient List, select Stephanie Brown (Room 304).
- Click on **Go to Nurses' Station** and then on **304** at the bottom of the screen.
- Click on **Patient Care** and complete a focused assessment of Stephanie Brown's neurological status by clicking on the appropriate body system categories (yellow buttons) and body system subcategories (green buttons).
- When you finish your assessment, click on **Leave the Floor**.
- From the Floor Menu, select **Look at Your Preceptor's Evaluations**.
- Next, click on **Examination Report** and review the feedback.

1. Reflect on your assessment skills. Did you miss any areas?

- To return to the Pediatrics Floor, click on **Return to Evaluations** and then on **Return to Menu**.
- From the Floor Menu, click on **Restart the Program**.
- Sign in to work on the Pediatrics Floor for Period of Care 2.
- From the Patient List, select Stephanie Brown (Room 304).
- Click on **Go to Nurses' Station** and then on **304** at the bottom of the screen.
- Click on **Patient Care** and then on **Nurse-Client Interactions**.
- Select and view the video titled **1120: Preventing Spread of Disease**. (*Note:* Check the virtual clock to see whether enough time has elapsed. You can use the fast-forward feature to advance the time by 2-minute intervals if the video is not yet available. Then click again on **Patient Care** and **Nurse-Client Interactions** to refresh the screen.)

2. CDC guidelines require standard precautions for all types of meningitis, as well as droplet precautions for certain types. What else must be done to effectively implement droplet precautions? (*Hint:* Refer to Appendix A in your textbook: Standard Precautions and Transmission-Based Isolation Precautions.)

3. The above guidelines are implemented immediately and kept in place until 24 hours after antibiotics have been started. Why?

4. When planning to administer antibiotics to the patient with meningitis, the nurse knows that:
   a. antibiotics must be administered before the cultures are obtained.
   b. antibiotics must be administered after the cultures are obtained.
   c. antibiotics must be administered after the culture results are completed.

5. What type of infection-prevention technique best describes the actions of the nurse in the video?
   a. Respiratory isolation
   b. Reverse isolation
   c. Enteric isolation
   d. Universal precautions

6. Suppose you see that Stephanie Brown's mother is not wearing a mask. When you ask her about this, she says she doesn't need to do anything special because she never leaves her daughter's room. How would you respond?

7. Every time you walk into the room with your mask on, Stephanie Brown starts to scream. This behavior occurs even when you have observed her through the window quietly playing with her mother before you come in the room. What is going on, and how might you respond?

- Again, click on **Patient Care** and then on **Nurse-Client Interactions**.
- Select and view the video titled **1145: Teaching—Disease Sequelae**. (*Note:* Check the virtual clock to see whether enough time has elapsed. You can use the fast-forward feature to advance the time by 2-minute intervals if the video is not yet available. Then click again on **Patient Care** and **Nurse-Client Interactions** to refresh the screen.)

8. The charge nurse tells you to take care when entering Stephanie Brown's room and when working with her. She also says to keep stimulation to a minimum. What does she mean, and how do you specifically need to behave?

- Click on **Chart** and then on **304**.
- Click on **Physician's Orders**.

9. Is Stephanie Brown on any treatment or medication that may contribute to permanent injury?

10. Review Stephanie Brown's IV orders. Calculate the total volume for 24 hours.

- Click on **Return to Room 304**.
- Next, click on **Leave the Floor** and then on **Restart the Program**.
- Sign in to work on the Pediatrics Floor for Period of Care 3.
- From the Patient List, select Stephanie Brown (Room 304).
- Click on **Go to Nurses' Station** and then on **304** at the bottom of the screen to go to Stephanie Brown's room.
- Click on **Patient Care** and then on **Nurse-Client Interactions**.
- Select and view the video titled **1510: Nurse-Patient Communication**. (*Note:* Check the virtual clock to see whether enough time has elapsed. You can use the fast-forward feature to advance the time by 2-minute intervals if the video is not yet available. Then click again on **Patient Care** and **Nurse-Client Interactions** to refresh the screen.)

11. What is the nurse's assessment and decision in the video?

12. The nurse explains to Stephanie Brown that she is going to apply a local anesthetic. What is a more age-appropriate way of saying this?

13. What anesthetic drug is being used? How is it used in order to be most effective? (*Hint:* See Chapter 22 in your textbook.)

14. Note the nurse's interaction with Stephanie Brown and her mother. Why is Stephanie Brown, who is only 3 years old, included in the explanation?

15. At Stephanie Brown's age, how might she perceive her hospital experience? How might she perceive the nurse?

16. How might the mother's behavior affect Stephanie Brown's perceptions?

17. From a developmental perspective, what are major fears of children in Stephanie Brown's age group? What behaviors might the child display?

18. What strategies can you use to promote a more positive experience for Stephanie Brown?

Caring for a Young Child with Cerebral Palsy

Reading Assignment: An Overview of Growth, Development, and Nutrition (Chapter 15)
The Toddler (Chapter 17)
The Preschool Child (Chapter 18)
The Child with a Sensory or Neurological Condition (Chapter 23)

Patient: Stephanie Brown, Pediatrics Floor, Room 304

Objectives:

1. Describe the behaviors and problems associated with the most common types of cerebral palsy.
2. Discuss a range of precipitating factors associated with cerebral palsy.
3. Explain the importance of early diagnosis and treatment to the child's optimal level of function.
4. Discuss the nursing care needs of a child with cerebral palsy.

Completing this lesson will help you gain an appreciation of the challenges associated with caring for a child who has cerebral palsy—both for parents and for the nurse. You will also explore the issue of encountering cerebral palsy as a condition that coexists with other health problems, the latter being the reason for hospitalization or other health care encounter. You will be working with Stephanie Brown in Room 304.

Exercise 1

Writing Activity

20 minutes

1. When children are hospitalized for an acute illness, you may find that they also have another disability or chronic illness that could have an effect on the hospitalization or on your care. Think about how you would provide care in such a situation. How do you get information? Who is in charge? Should you involve parents in the same ways you normally do?

2. Consider ideas for teaching parents to promote their child's self-esteem as the child progresses through the stage of initiative versus guilt. What strategies might you suggest?

3. Which factors could potentially cause cerebral palsy? Select all that apply.

_____ Premature birth

_____ Severe maternal hyperglycemia

_____ Existing prenatal brain abnormalities

_____ Exposure to maternal infections

_____ Shaken baby syndrome

4. Describe cerebral palsy.

5. Indicate whether each of the following statements is true or false.

a. _____ Cerebral palsy may either start in infancy or while in utero.

b. _____ Cerebral palsy will cause epilepsy.

6. What types of fine and gross motor functions may be affected by cerebral palsy?

Exercise 2

Virtual Hospital Activity

30 minutes

- Sign in to work at Pacific View Regional Hospital on the Pediatrics Floor for Period of Care 1. (*Note:* If you are already in the virtual hospital from a previous exercise, click on **Leave the Floor** and then on **Restart the Program** to get to the sign-in window.)
- From the Patient List, select Stephanie Brown (Room 304).
- Click on **Get Report** and read the Clinical Report.
- Click on **Go to Nurses' Station** and then on **304** at the bottom of the screen to go to Stephanie Brown's room.
- Click on **Patient Care** and perform a focused assessment by clicking on the body system categories (yellow buttons) and the body system subcategories (green buttons).

1. Based on your assessment of Stephanie Brown, list any behavioral responses she demonstrates that are associated with cerebral palsy.

2. In addition to the symptoms manifested by Stephanie Brown, the nurse must recognize that cerebral palsy may be suspected if which issues are noted? Select all that apply.

_____ Delayed achievement of milestones

_____ Psychosocial immaturity

_____ Feeding problems

_____ Diminished Moro reflex

_____ Abnormal fatigue with activity

- Click on **Chart** and then on **304**.
- Click on the **History and Physical** tab.

3. Review Stephanie Brown's history. What factor(s) might have contributed to her cerebral palsy?

4. Think about nursing admissions procedures. What additional information would be especially important to have?

- Click on **Return to Room 304**.
- Click on **Patient Care** and then on **Nurse-Client Interactions**.
- Select and view the video titled **0750: Caring for the Child with CP**. (*Note:* Check the virtual clock to see whether enough time has elapsed. You can use the fast-forward feature to advance the time by 2-minute intervals if the video is not yet available. Then click again on **Patient Care** and **Nurse-Client Interactions** to refresh the screen.)

5. What should the nurse be doing as she listens to the mother explain the problems that Stephanie Brown has associated with cerebral palsy?

6. Should the nurse be supportive of Stephanie Brown's mother implementing the treatments and strategies she uses at home in the hospital? Why or why not?

7. For what problem is Stephanie Brown at risk during her hospitalization? (*Hint:* You will need to consider Stephanie Brown's developmental age.)

- Click on **Chart** and then on **304**.
- Click on the **Nursing Admission** tab and review for data about Stephanie Brown's development.

8. Hospitalization can still be a time of growth. Explore which developmental tasks Stephanie Brown has achieved and which she has not. Comment on her development.

9. The developmental stage for Stephanie Brown at this age is:
   a. trust versus mistrust.
   b. autonomy versus shame and doubt.
   c. ego integrity versus despair.
   d. initiative versus guilt.

10. This is a good opportunity to explore Stephanie Brown's development further. One assessment tool that can be used is the Denver Developmental Screening Test II (DDST-II).
    Identify the areas assessed on this test.

11. Parents often express concern about their child's performance when the DDST II is used. Explain the purpose of this test and discuss what a screening test is.

Exercise 3

Virtual Hospital Activity

30 minutes

- Sign in to work at Pacific View Regional Hospital on the Pediatrics Floor for Period of Care 3. (*Note:* If you are already in the virtual hospital from a previous exercise, click on **Leave the Floor** and then on **Restart the Program** to get to the sign-in window.)
- From the Patient List, select Stephanie Brown (Room 304).
- Click on **Get Report** and read the Clinical Report.
- Click on **Go to Nurses' Station**.
- Click on **Chart** and then on **304**.
- Review Stephanie Brown's records, in particular her **History and Physical**.

1. Match each type of cerebral palsy with its description.

	Type		**Description**
_____	Spastic	a.	Rigid flexor and extensor muscles; tremors
_____	Dyskinetic/athetoid	b.	Increased deep tendon reflexes, hypertonia, flexion, and scissors gait
_____	Ataxic	c.	Slow, writhing, uncontrolled, and involuntary movements
_____	Mixed	d.	Loss of coordination, equilibrium, and kinesthetic sense

2. What type of cerebral palsy does Stephanie Brown have? What are the signs that she manifests?

3. Cerebral palsy can have an impact on many aspects of a child's life. A number of problems can be associated with the behaviors the child manifests. What are some of these problems? (*Note:* Make sure that at least one is a psychosocial concern.)

4. If Stephanie Brown's mother expresses guilt over her daughter's condition and states that she knows now that she did some things that may have contributed to the condition, how would you respond?

5. Stephanie Brown's mother asks you whether you see signs of mental retardation in her daughter. She is worried that this will develop as Stephanie Brown's disease progresses. Which of the following responses to her is most appropriate?
   a. "It is still a little early for the signs of retardation to develop."
   b. "Since she does not have obvious signs of retardation yet, she will be fine."
   c. "Cerebral palsy does not cause mental retardation."
   d. "You should have a consultation with a physician."

- Click on **Return to Nurses' Station** and then on **304** at the bottom of the screen.
- Click on **Patient Care** and then on **Nurse-Client Interactions**.
- Select and view the video titled **1530: Preventive Measures**. (*Note:* Check the virtual clock to see whether enough time has elapsed. You can use the fast-forward feature to advance the time by 2-minute intervals if the video is not yet available. Then click again on **Patient Care** and **Nurse-Client Interactions** to refresh the screen.)

6. Why does Stephanie Brown require heel cord stretching?

7. What other preventive measures have been integrated into Stephanie Brown's regimen to prevent complications associated with cerebral palsy?

8. What is the role of the nurse in regard to supporting the mother's implementation of these measures?

9. Explain why nutrition is so important for the child who has cerebral palsy.

Caring for a School-Age Child with Diabetes Mellitus

Reading Assignment: The School-Age Child (Chapter 19)
The Child with a Metabolic Condition (Chapter 31)

Patient: George Gonzalez, Pediatrics Floor, Room 301

Objectives:

1. Review the pathophysiology of diabetes mellitus.
2. Compare and contrast type 1 and type 2 diabetes.
3. Explain the role of insulin in the metabolism of foods.
4. Explain the classic signs of diabetes: polyuria, polydipsia, and polyphagia.
5. Discuss management and nursing responsibilities for insulin therapy, diet, exercise, and blood glucose monitoring.
6. Contrast hypoglycemia and hyperglycemia with regard to causes, signs and symptoms, and management.
7. Explain diabetic ketoacidosis and discuss its management and nursing care.
8. Discuss the impact of growth and development on diabetes.

Most likely, you have already learned about diabetes and have a basic understanding of the disease and its problems. In this lesson you will work with 11-year-old George Gonzalez. You will learn about diabetes in children by considering problems and nursing care for George Gonzalez's illness. In doing so, you will need to apply principles of growth and development. Although teaching may be addressed in this lesson, more specifics on the learning needs for the child and the family, along with the nurse's responsibilities, will be found in the next lesson.

Exercise 1

Writing Activity

30 minutes

The assumption is that you have encountered information about diabetes mellitus in your educational experience. Let's begin by going over some key points. (*Hint:* If you run across something with which you are unfamiliar, you may need to take the time to do a little more review.)

1. Describe diabetes mellitus.

2. Differentiate between type 1 and type 2 diabetes mellitus by matching each of the following characteristics to its corresponding type of diabetes mellitus.

Characteristic	Type of Diabetes Mellitus
_____ Most common endocrine disease in children	a. Type 1 diabetes mellitus
_____ Results from destruction of pancreatic beta cells	b. Type 2 diabetes mellitus
_____ Cells unable to use insulin	
_____ Genetic predisposition	
_____ Pancreas unable to produce insulin	
_____ Commonly characterized by obesity	
_____ Prone to ketosis	
_____ Also called noninsulin-dependent diabetes mellitus	
_____ Also called insulin-dependent diabetes mellitus	

3. What symptoms might a child have at the time that diabetes is diagnosed? (*Hint:* Be sure to consider growth and development in your discussion.)

4. Which are signs of hyperglycemia? Select all that apply.

_____ Decrease in urination

_____ Increased thirst

_____ Nervous energy

_____ Weight gain

_____ Dehydration

_____ Disorientation

_____ Drowsiness

_____ Hunger

_____ Tachycardia

5. List three factors that are often included in the management of hyperglycemia.

6. Discuss the relationship between exercise and insulin needs.

7. When planning the dietary needs of a child with diabetes, what factor is used to determine caloric needs?

8. The dietary intake for a child with diabetes should consist of _____ % carbohydrates, _____ % protein,

and _____ % fats.

9. What are the signs of hypoglycemia?

10. How is hypoglycemia managed?

11. What is HbA1C? Explain its use as a diagnostic and monitoring tool.

12. A combination of a short-acting and an intermediate-acting insulin is often ordered for patients with diabetes. Match each characteristic with its corresponding type of insulin. (*Hint:* See Table 31-6 in your textbook.)

Characteristic	Type of Insulin
_____ Onset of 30 to 60 minutes	a. Regular
_____ Onset of 1 to 2 hours	b. NPH
_____ Peak at 4 to 12 hours	c. Insulin glargine
_____ Peak at 2 to 5 hours	d. Insulin lispro
_____ Duration of 5 to 8 hours	
_____ Duration of 14 to 24 hours	
_____ Onset of 1 hour	
_____ Duration of 3 to 5 hours	

13. Based on the above information, at what time of day would a person who receives NPH insulin in the morning be at greatest risk for a hypoglycemic episode?
    a. Mid-morning
    b. Mid-afternoon
    c. After dinner
    d. During the night

Exercise 2

Virtual Hospital Activity

60 minutes

- Sign in to work at Pacific View Regional Hospital on the Pediatrics Floor for Period of Care 1. (*Note:* If you are already in the virtual hospital from another exercise, click on **Leave the Floor** and then on **Restart the Program** to get to the sign-in window.)
- From the patient List, select George Gonzalez (Room 301).
- Click on **Go to Nurses' Station**.
- Click on **Chart** and then on **301**.
- Click on the **Emergency Department** tab and review this record.

1. George Gonzalez has been admitted with a diagnosis of diabetic ketoacidosis (DKA). What does this mean?

2. What signs and symptoms did George Gonzalez manifest on admission to the Emergency Department? Is there a known precipitating factor? What are *possible* precipitating factors of DKA?

3. What will be the focus of care for the first portion of George Gonzalez's hospitalization for DKA?

4. IV insulin is used to manage DKA. What type of insulin may be administered by way of an IV?
   a. Lantus
   b. NPH
   c. Regular
   d. Lispro

5. Identify any nursing concerns associated with IV administration of insulin.

• Continue reviewing the **Emergency Department** record and look for a pattern in George Gonzalez's blood glucose levels.
• Click on **Laboratory Reports** and review the results for glucose.

6. What was George Gonzalez's blood glucose level on admission to the Emergency Department? What was it after a period of IV therapy with insulin?

- Click on the **History and Physical** tab and review the information given.

7. Why was George Gonzalez at an increased risk for development of diabetes mellitus?

8. What ongoing assessments do you need to make when caring for George Gonzalez?

9. Even though blood glucose monitors are used almost exclusively, why is urine testing still performed when DKA is the diagnosis?

- Click on **Return to Nurses' Station**.
- Click on **301** at the bottom of the screen.
- Click on **Patient Care** and then on **Nurse-Client Interactions**.
- Select and view the video titled **0730: Supervision—Glucose Testing**. (*Note:* Check the virtual clock to see whether enough time has elapsed. You can use the fast-forward feature to advance the time by 2-minute intervals if the video is not yet available. Then click again on **Patient Care** and **Nurse-Client Interactions** to refresh the screen.)

10. What did the nurse do that facilitated George Gonzalez's honesty about how he tests and how he feels about it?

11. What is the nurse trying to accomplish when she asks George Gonzalez to do his own fingerstick? (*Hint:* Consider the developmental tasks of a school-age child.)

12. How might George Gonzalez's age and interests affect his compliance with treatment?

- Click on **Return to Nurses' Station**.
- Click on **301** at the bottom of the screen.
- Click **Patient Care** and then on **Nurse-Client Interactions**.
- Select and view the video titled **0745: Self-Administering Insulin**. (*Note:* Check the virtual clock to see whether enough time has elapsed. You can use the fast-forward feature to advance the time by 2-minute intervals if the video is not yet available. Then click again on **Patient Care** and **Nurse-Client Interactions** to refresh the screen.)

13. What positive actions does the nurse take as she observes George Gonzalez give himself his injection?

George Gonzalez needs insulin. Before going to the Medication Room, complete any necessary assessments.

- Click on **MAR** to check the order for insulin and then click on **Return to Room 301**.
- Click on **Medication Room** at the bottom of the screen.
- Using the six rights, prepare the correct dose of insulin for George Gonzalez. When you have prepared the medication, return to the patient's room and administer it, again following the six rights. (*Hint:* Try to perform these steps on your own. If you need help, refer to pages 24-28 and 35-39 in the **Getting Started** section of this workbook.)
- After administering the insulin, click on **Leave the Floor** and then on **Look at Your Preceptor's Evaluations**.
- Next, click on **Medication Scorecard** and review the feedback.

14. Do you need to do anything differently to satisfactorily complete the procedure? If so, explain.

- Click on **Return to Evaluations** and then on **Return to Menu**.
- Click on **Restart the Program**.
- Sign in to work on the Pediatrics Floor for Period of Care 1.
- From the Patient List, select George Gonzalez (Room 301).
- Click on **Go to Nurses' Station**.
- Click on **Chart** and then on **301**.
- Click on the **Physician's Orders** tab. Find the order for George Gonzalez's morning dose of insulin.

15. Using this insulin order, describe the steps for drawing up two different insulins into one syringe.

16. Why is short-acting insulin always drawn up first?

17. How should George Gonzalez be advised to rotate injection sites?

Let's jump ahead in virtual time to review and reinforce your insulin administrations skills.

- Click on **Return to Nurses' Station**, **Leave the Floor**, and **Restart the Program**.
- Sign in to work on the Pediatrics Floor for Period of Care 2.
- From the Patient List, select George Gonzalez (Room 301).
- Click on **Go to Nurses' Station**.
- Once again, prepare and administer George Gonzalez's morning dose of insulin. Using the six rights, be sure to check the order, as well as George Gonzalez's current blood glucose level. Perform the proper identification checks before giving the medication.
- After administering the insulin, check your performance by reviewing the preceptor's **Medication Scorecard**.

18. Reflect on your performance. Consider the actual practice you may need in order to feel comfortable with this skill.

19. List the learning needs of patients newly diagnosed with diabetes.

20. Which of the above learning needs do George Gonzalez and his family currently have?

- To return to the floor, click on **Return to Evaluations**, **Return to Menu**, and **Restart the Program**.
- Sign in to work on the Pediatrics Floor, again for Period of Care 2.
- From the Patient List, select George Gonzalez (Room 301).
- Click on **Go to Nurses' Station** and then on **301** at the bottom of the screen.
- Click on **Patient Care** and then on **Nurse-Client Interactions**.
- Select and view the video titled **1115: Teaching—Disease Process**. (*Note:* Check the virtual clock to see whether enough time has elapsed. You can use the fast-forward feature to advance the time by 2-minute intervals if the video is not yet available. Then click again on **Patient Care** and **Nurse-Client Interactions** to refresh the screen.)

21. What are the sequelae of untreated or poorly managed diabetes? Explain why these occur.

Exercise 3

Writing Activity

5 minutes

1. What are some approaches for responding to the learning needs of children such as George Gonzalez?

2. Compare and contrast two or more websites designed for individuals with diabetes and their families. Write about each website's target audience, ease of use, and appropriateness for patients with diabetes and their families. You may do a search and select your own websites or choose from the following established sites:
   - *www.diabetes.org*
   - *www.jdrf.org*
   - *www.niddk.nih.gov*

Supporting the Child with Diabetes and His Family While They Learn Self-Care

Reading Assignment: The Toddler (Chapter 17)
The Preschool Child (Chapter 18)
The School-Age Child (Chapter 19)
The Adolescent (Chapter 20)
The Child with a Metabolic Condition (Chapter 31)

Patient: George Gonzalez, Pediatrics Floor, Room 301

Objectives:

1. Identify the learning needs of a child newly diagnosed with diabetes mellitus.
2. Construct a developmentally appropriate plan for teaching a child independence with care of diabetes.
3. Explore the need for information, readiness, capability, and motivation as significant factors in the teaching-learning process.
4. Differentiate between the roles of the child and the parent in managing the child's diabetes.

In this lesson you will focus on the teaching aspect in the care of the child with diabetes. You will consider learning needs according to the child's developmental stage and parental responsibilities, along with the dynamic nature of supervision and self-care. You may need to review developmental issues associated with various age groups. You may also need to review the teaching-learning process since you will be applying these principles throughout your work.

Exercise 1

Writing Activity

45 minutes

1. When determining the teaching needs of a child with diabetes and the child's family, which factors should be given consideration? Select all that apply.

    _____ Children must have a cognitive understanding of the skills before the skills are taught by the nurse.

    _____ Motor skill proficiency precedes cognitive awareness of related information.

    _____ The nurse will need to assess fine motor development before teaching the child related skills such as insulin administration and blood glucose monitoring.

    _____ The parents may be performing some of the care skills until the child is fully capable.

2. What are the roles and responsibilities of the family in care?

3. When working with the parents of a toddler diagnosed with diabetes, what age-appropriate strategies may be recommended by the nurse?
    a. Allowing broad choices to the child to promote involvement
    b. Discouraging rituals to reduce boredom with care interventions
    c. Structuring care interventions to eliminate the need for the child to participate
    d. Using distraction when implementing painful interventions

4. The nurse is observing the parents of a preschool-age child. When administering insulin, which strategy is most effective?
    a. Offering the child a toy or special privilege if the child begins to cry during the therapy
    b. Offering the child a toy or special privilege after the procedure with the condition that the child behaves during the therapy
    c. Avoiding the use of rewards when administering the treatments
    d. Offering toys or special privileges before the initiation of therapies that are to be awarded after the treatments are completed

5. What are some care issues for the preschool-age child with diabetes? What might you suggest to parents? (*Hint:* Refer to Chapter 18 in your textbook.)

6. What are some care issues if the child with diabetes is of school-age? What might you suggest to parents? (*Hint:* Refer to Chapter 19 in your textbook.)

7. What are some care issues if the child with diabetes is an adolescent? What might you suggest to parents? (*Hint:* Refer to Chapter 20 in your textbook.)

8. You are working with a family whose child was recently diagnosed with diabetes. List several areas that you would want to discuss about diabetes in general.

9. The nurse has determined that a child diagnosed with diabetes is experiencing the "honeymoon" phase of the disease. What information should be provided to the parents? Select all that apply.

_____   Improvements in the child's condition will usually last for several months.

_____   This phase is most common in individuals with type 2 diabetes mellitus.

_____   Insulin needs will decrease during this phase of the disease.

_____   Close monitoring of the child's condition is needed during this time.

_____   It is common for the child to begin to feel better during this phase of the disease.

10. What would you do to explain the relationships among food, exercise, and insulin in a way that would be meaningful to parents?

11. Health maintenance and regular visits with health care providers are important, even when the child is doing well. Discuss the issue of who (parent, child, or both) should be in attendance at an office visit.

12. Describe potential barriers to providing optimal outpatient care for the child with diabetes and the child's family.

13. You are assisting a nurse who is working with the mother of a child newly diagnosed with diabetes. You observe the teary-eyed parent with an orange and a syringe. How would you respond?

14. Discuss the advantages of diabetes groups or camps for children.

Exercise 2

Virtual Hospital Activity

30 minutes

- Sign in to work at Pacific View Regional Hospital on the Pediatrics Floor for Period of Care 1. (*Note:* If you are already in the virtual hospital from a previous exercise, click on **Leave the Floor** and then on **Restart the Program** to get to the sign-in window.)
- From the Patient List, select George Gonzalez (Room 301).
- Click on **Go to Nurses' Station** and then on **301** at the bottom of the screen.
- Click on **Patient Care** and then on **Nurse-Client Interactions**.
- Select and view the video titled **0730: Supervision—Glucose Testing**. (*Note:* Check the virtual clock to see whether enough time has elapsed. You can use the fast-forward feature to advance the time by 2-minute intervals if the video is not yet available. Then click again on **Patient Care** and **Nurse-Client Interactions** to refresh the screen.)

1. Is George Gonzalez physically capable of being responsible for his own blood glucose testing? Comment on his skill and knowledge level for glucose testing.

2. What are some possible reasons that George Gonzalez may be noncompliant with blood glucose testing?

3. What effective actions does the nurse take? What other interventions can be offered?

4. Identify information that is necessary for families to understand about insulin.

5. Identify effective techniques to use for teaching insulin administration to parents and children. Provide rationales where appropriate.

6. Which are potential barriers to learning insulin injection techniques? Select all that apply.

_____ Level of growth and development

_____ Fear of needles

_____ Cognitive deficits

_____ Lack of self discipline

_____ Misinformation about the treatment plan

7. List several issues associated with site selection and rotation that should be discussed with George Gonzalez and his family.

8. How should site selection be considered in relation to absorption?

- Click on **Patient Care** and then on **Nurse-Client Interactions**.
- Select and view the video titled **0745: Self-Administering Insulin**. (*Note:* Check the virtual clock to see whether enough time has elapsed. You can use the fast-forward feature to advance the time by 2-minute intervals if the video is not yet available. Then click again on **Patient Care** and **Nurse-Client Interactions** to refresh the screen.)

9. Evaluate George Gonzalez's performance and comment on anything else you need to do with him to improve his performance.

Exercise 3

Virtual Hospital Activity

30 minutes

- Sign in to work at Pacific View Regional Hospital on the Pediatrics Floor for Period of Care 2. (*Note:* If you are already in the virtual hospital from a previous exercise, click on **Leave the Floor** and then on **Restart the Program** to get to the sign-in window.)
- From the Patient List, select George Gonzalez (Room 301).
- Click on **Go to Nurses' Station** and then on **301** at the bottom of the screen.
- Click on **Patient Care** and then on **Nurse-Client Interactions**.
- Select and view the video titled **1115: Teaching—Disease Process**. (*Note:* Check the virtual clock to see whether enough time has elapsed. You can use the fast-forward feature to advance the time by 2-minute intervals if the video is not yet available. Then click again on **Patient Care** and **Nurse-Client Interactions** to refresh the screen.)

1. Evaluate George Gonzalez's understanding of his condition and management of hypoglycemia.

2. What is his mother's level of understanding?

3. Given the responses of George Gonzalez and his mother, is there a need for teaching in this area? If so, what type of teaching needs to be done?

- Click again on **Patient Care** and then on **Nurse-Client Interactions**.
- Select and view the video titled **1130: Teaching—Managing Symptoms**. (*Note:* Check the virtual clock to see whether enough time has elapsed. You can use the fast-forward feature to advance the time by 2-minute intervals if the video is not yet available. Then click again on **Patient Care** and **Nurse-Client Interactions** to refresh the screen.)

4. Do you think George Gonzalez and his mother understand the concept of managing symptoms? Explain your answer.

5. What should the nurse do based on this assessment of George Gonzalez and his mother's level of understanding?

6. Nothing has been said about record keeping. What would you suggest?

Let's jump ahead in virtual time to observe a nurse-patient interaction that occurs later in the day.

- Click on **Leave the Floor** and then **Restart the Program**.
- Sign in to work at Pacific View Regional Hospital on the Pediatrics Floor for Period of Care 3.
- From the Patient List, select George Gonzalez (Room 301).
- Click on **Go to Nurses' Station** and then on **301** at the bottom of the screen.
- Click on **Patient Care** and then on **Nurse-Client Interactions**.
- Select and view the video titled **1500: Teaching—Diabetic Diet**. (*Note:* Check the virtual clock to see whether enough time has elapsed. You can use the fast-forward feature to advance the time by 2-minute intervals if the video is not yet available. Then click again on **Patient Care** and **Nurse-Client Interactions** to refresh the screen.)

7. What is George Gonzalez's diet order? What are the recommendations of the dietitian?

8. Evaluate the nurse's teaching with regard to diet. What did she do well? What could she have explained better?

9. Is there anything that the nurse should pursue with George Gonzalez's mother?

- Click on **Patient Care** and then on **Nurse-Client Interactions**.
- Select and view the video titled **1535: Teaching—Effects of Exercise**. (*Note:* Check the virtual clock to see whether enough time has elapsed. You can use the fast-forward feature to advance the time by 2-minute intervals if the video is not yet available. Then click again on **Patient Care** and **Nurse-Client Interactions** to refresh the screen.)

10. Discuss the effects of physical activity on blood glucose levels. Consider times of day when George Gonzalez might have more activity than others.

11. What should George Gonzalez be advised to do in relation to activity?

12. Based on the potential complications discussed in question 10, do you think it would be better if George Gonzalez did not exercise? Explain your response. (*Hint:* Be sure to consider growth and development as a factor.)

Caring for a Teen with an Eating Disorder

Reading Assignment: The Adolescent (Chapter 20)
The Child with an Emotional or Behavioral Condition (Chapter 33)

Patient: Tiffany Sheldon, Pediatrics Floor, Room 305

Objectives:

1. Compare and contrast the description, etiology, and typical behaviors associated with anorexia nervosa and bulimia nervosa.
2. Discuss the physiological impacts of anorexia nervosa and bulimia nervosa.
3. Discuss the multidisciplinary approach necessary for treatment of eating disorders.
4. Explore the challenges of providing nursing care for patients with anorexia nervosa or bulimia nervosa.

In this lesson you will explore a variety of challenges associated with caring for a teen with an eating disorder. You will care for Tiffany Sheldon, a 14-year-old female with a history of eight admissions in the past 2 years for complications associated with anorexia nervosa. You will learn that helping a patient manage an eating disorder requires intensive multidisciplinary effort.

Note: Generally, when the facilities are available, patients with eating disorders are transferred to the Eating Disorders Unit, where professionals are highly skilled and experienced with this area of care. However, this may not be the case in all settings; thus all nurses need to be aware of the problems, the risks, and the usual approaches to treatment of eating disorders. You will have accomplished this by completing this lesson.

Exercise 1

Writing Activity

20 minutes

1. Match each characteristic listed below with its corresponding eating disorder—anorexia nervosa, bulimia nervosa, or both. (*Hint:* Although some characteristics may seem to overlap, most are usually associated more closely with one problem rather than the other. In those cases, choose the problem most closely associated with the characteristic.)

Characteristic	**Type of Eating Disorder**
_____ Deliberate refusal of food to maintain body weight	a. Anorexia nervosa
_____ Recurrent episodes of binging and a sense of loss of control	b. Bulimia nervosa
_____ Misuse of laxatives and/or diuretics	c. Both anorexia and bulimia
_____ Amenorrhea	
_____ Overconcern with body image, though not distorted	
_____ Body image that is contrary to reality	
_____ Ritualistic eating pattern	
_____ Binge eating and purging	
_____ Muscle wasting, dull and brittle hair, presence of lanugo	
_____ Electrolyte imbalance	
_____ Tooth erosion	
_____ Self-induced vomiting	
_____ Risk factor: participation in sports, dance, or gymnastics	
_____ Cardiac arrhythmias	
_____ Excessive exercise	
_____ Excessive influence of body weight on self-evaluation	
_____ History of family dysfunction	
_____ Weight of less than 85% of what is expected	

2. Give an example of an eating pattern that might be found in a person with anorexia nervosa. What often underlies such behavior?

3. When reviewing the family history of a client diagnosed with anorexia nervosa, which characteristic may be noted?
   a. Permissive parenting styles
   b. Rigid, rule-filled family life
   c. Low socioeconomic status
   d. Relaxed approach to discipline

4. How is it believed that family function and culture play into the problem of eating disorders?

5. What are some secondary gains achieved through eating disorders? (*Hint:* Secondary gains are perceived benefits other than weight loss that the patient gets from his or her disease.)

_____ Attention

_____ Envy of others

_____ Sense of self satisfaction

_____ Increase in self-confidence

_____ Increased control over others

6. Nurses in schools or other community settings may play several roles with teens who have anorexia nervosa. Discuss one of the primary roles.

7. Assume that you are working in a community setting and a teen says to you, "I have to tell you something, but you can't tell anyone." What response is the most appropriate?
   a. "Of course, what you tell me will be kept in the strictest of confidence."
   b. "If you share things with me that indicate you or your health is at risk, I may have to report it."
   c. "The physician is the only one who can assure you complete confidentiality."
   d. "As long as what you share does not involve child abuse, I can keep it secret."

Exercise 2

Virtual Hospital Activity

30 minutes

- Sign in to work at Pacific View Regional Hospital on the Pediatrics Floor for Period of Care 1. (*Note:* If you are already in the virtual hospital from a previous exercise, click on **Leave the Floor** and then on **Restart the Program** to get to the sign-in window.)
- From the Patient List, select Tiffany Sheldon (Room 305).
- Click on **Go to Nurses' Station**.
- Click on **Chart** and then on **305**.
- Click on and review the **Nursing Admission** and the **History and Physical**.

1. What in Tiffany Sheldon's history is indicative of her diagnosis of anorexia nervosa?

- Click on **Return to Nurses' Station** and then on **305** at the bottom of the screen.
- Click on **Patient Care** and complete a head-to-toe assessment, noting data that are consistent with anorexia nervosa.
- Click on **Patient Care** and then on **Nurse-Client Interactions**.
- Select and view the video titled **0730: Initial Assessment**. (*Note:* Check the virtual clock to see whether enough time has elapsed. You can use the fast-forward feature to advance the time by 2-minute intervals if the video is not yet available. Then click again on **Patient Care** and **Nurse-Client Interactions** to refresh the screen.)

2. Tiffany Sheldon has been described as having a flat affect, being withdrawn, and avoiding eye contact. How would you describe her behavior at the time of this video interaction?

3. What is the most effective form of communication to use with Tiffany Sheldon?

4. Is there anything in the video that you need to report? If so, what?

- Again, click on **Patient Care** and then on **Nurse-Client Interactions**.
- Select and view the video titled **0800: Coordinating Care**. (*Note:* Check the virtual clock to see whether enough time has elapsed. You can use the fast-forward feature to advance the time by 2-minute intervals if the video is not yet available. Then click again on **Patient Care** and **Nurse-Client Interactions** to refresh the screen.)

5. What emotion would you expect Tiffany Sheldon to express if she were told that she would be seen by an Eating Disorders Team?
   a. Anger
   b. Acceptance
   c. Excitement
   d. Casual interest

6. What is the nurse's role in identifying and/or coordinating care and services that Tiffany Sheldon requires during her inpatient stay?

Exercise 3

Virtual Hospital Activity

45 minutes

The first order of business with a patient who has anorexia nervosa is to correct any fluid and electrolyte imbalances. Keep this in mind as you work through this exercise.

- Sign in to work at Pacific View Regional Hospital on the Pediatrics Floor for Period of Care 1. (*Note:* If you are already in the virtual hospital from a previous exercise, click on **Leave the Floor** and then on **Restart the Program** to get to the sign-in window.)
- From the Patient List, select Tiffany Sheldon (Room 305).
- Click on **Go to Nurses' Station**.
- Click on **Chart** and then on **305**.
- Click on and review the **Physician's Orders** and the **Laboratory Reports**.

1. What do Tiffany Sheldon's lab results tell you about her fluid and electrolyte status? Report on the ones that give you specific information.

2. What is being done to assess for and manage Tiffany Sheldon's fluid and electrolyte imbalance?

3. List the objective assessment data that indicate Tiffany Sheldon is dehydrated.

4. Why is Tiffany Sheldon on a cardiac monitor?

5. Tiffany Sheldon is receiving IV fluid with potassium chloride added. What is the order? What are the nursing responsibilities before and during potassium administration?

6. You need to be familiar with care plans for common problems associated with anorexia nervosa. Work on the following problem.

 a. Identify a generic nursing diagnosis for hydration problems in patients with anorexia nervosa.

 b. Now rewrite your nursing diagnosis so that it accurately reflects Tiffany Sheldon's situation.

Next, begin thinking about how adequate caloric intake is achieved.

- Click on **Return to Nurse's Station** and then on **Leave the Floor**.
- From the Floor Menu, select **Restart the Program**.
- Sign in to work at Pacific View Regional Hospital on the Pediatrics Floor for Period of Care 2.
- From the Patient List, select Tiffany Sheldon (Room 305).
- Click on **Go to Nurses' Station** and then on **305** at the bottom of the screen.
- Click on **Patient Care** and then on **Nurse-Client Interactions**.
- Select and view the video titled **1115: Managing Anorexia Nervosa**. (*Note:* Check the virtual clock to see whether enough time has elapsed. You can use the fast-forward feature to advance the time by 2-minute intervals if the video is not yet available. Then click again on **Patient Care** and **Nurse-Client Interactions** to refresh the screen.)

7. Discuss the cultural beliefs and personal perceptions that influence the development of eating disorders. Consider both males and females in your discussion.

8. What is the value of an eating contract for Tiffany Sheldon?

9. What is the rationale for including diet orders as part of the eating contract?

10. Calculate Tiffany Sheldon's daily caloric needs.

- Once again, click on **Patient Care** and then on **Nurse-Client Interactions**.
- Select and view the video titled **1130: Monitoring Compliance**. (*Note:* Check the virtual clock to see whether enough time has elapsed. You can use the fast-forward feature to advance the time by 2-minute intervals if the video is not yet available. Then click again on **Patient Care** and **Nurse-Client Interactions** to refresh the screen.)

11. Why have the measures cited in the video been put into Tiffany Sheldon's eating contract?

12. What supportive interventions might the nurse provide to help Tiffany Sheldon remain compliant?

Now, consider the emotional aspects of Tiffany Sheldon's care.

- Click on **Leave the Floor** and then **Restart the Program**.
- Sign in to work at Pacific View Regional Hospital on the Pediatrics Floor for Period of Care 3.
- From the Patient List, select Tiffany Sheldon (Room 305).
- Click on **Go to Nurses' Station** and then on **305** at the bottom of the screen.
- Click on **Patient Care** and then on **Nurse-Client Interactions**.
- Select and view the video titled **1500: Relapse—Contributing Factors**. (*Note:* Check the virtual clock to see whether enough time has elapsed. You can use the fast-forward feature to advance the time by 2-minute intervals if the video is not yet available. Then click again on **Patient Care** and **Nurse-Client Interactions** to refresh the screen.)

13. What does Tiffany Sheldon say in regard to what has caused her relapse? What recent events, if any, may have contributed to her having an acute episode of her anorexia nervosa?

14. What did the psychiatrist do to effectively elicit Tiffany Sheldon's concerns?

- Click on **Patient Care** and then on **Nurse-Client Interactions**.
- Select and view the video titled **1530: Facilitating Success**. (*Note:* Check the virtual clock to see whether enough time has elapsed. You can use the fast-forward feature to advance the time by 2-minute intervals if the video is not yet available. Then click again on **Patient Care** and **Nurse-Client Interactions** to refresh the screen.)

15. What does Tiffany Sheldon say about her progress?

16. What multidimensional factors will contribute to Tiffany Sheldon's ability to comply with the eating contract that has been developed? What barriers may be present?

17. A patient with an eating disorder may not like the sensations associated with refeeding. Develop several strategies to help Tiffany Sheldon overcome barriers to the success of her treatment plan.

18. Let's assume that Tiffany Sheldon refuses to eat and her condition puts her at even greater health risk. The hospital is awaiting a court order for a feeding tube. Tiffany Sheldon will need to be restrained if the order is implemented. How would you handle this situation? What would be your responsibilities as a nurse? (*Hint:* You may want to refer to a fundamentals of nursing textbook.)

Emergency Care for a Child with Head Trauma

Reading Assignment: The Child's Experience of Hospitalization (Chapter 21)
The Child with a Sensory or Neurological Condition (Chapter 23)

Patient: Tommy Douglas, Pediatrics Floor, Room 302

Objectives:

1. Consider factors that may create a stressful environment in emergency care.
2. Discuss nursing interventions supportive to the child and family who are experiencing emergency care.
3. Discuss the concept of "across the room" assessment and priority setting for a child in the Emergency Department.
4. Explore the implications of growth and development in emergency care.
5. Explore medications frequently used in traumatic emergency situations.
6. Identify priority concerns related to head injury.

In this lesson you will explore the role of the nurse in caring for a child in an emergency situation. More often than not, the priority needs of the child will be physiological, but the psychosocial care for family cannot be ignored. Parents have many support needs that sometimes are pushed aside during the acute phase of the visit. You will learn general strategies for dealing with such issues. You will be working with 6-year-old Tommy Douglas, who has arrived in the Emergency Department after a blunt trauma injury.

Exercise 1

Writing Activity

20 minutes

1. List and explain several factors that can contribute to a stressful environment for a child who is brought to the Emergency Department after a traumatic event.

2. For each of the factors you listed above, develop a nursing intervention to minimize stress. If you have had experience in such an environment (even during an observation), you have an opportunity to be creative here.

3. What do you think is meant by the notion of "assessment from across the room"? Identify some assessments that can be made in this manner.

4. Rank the following care items in order of priority, with 1 indicating the highest-priority care item and 7 indicating the lowest-priority care item.

_____ Trauma scoring

_____ Assessment of child's coping

_____ Circulatory assessment

_____ History of injury

_____ Breathing assessment

_____ Airway assessment

_____ Signs of other injury

5. Which factors are the top two concerns of children who are confronted with emergency care?

_____ Fear of body intrusion

_____ Fear of the unknown

_____ Pain

_____ Separation

_____ Unfamiliar environment

6. Parents and caregivers need a great deal of support. Nurses need to be able to anticipate fears and anxieties in order to craft careful communication to elicit and respond to concerns. What are some common fears or concerns parents have when their child is brought to the Emergency Department?

7. Parents may feel pushed aside in the Emergency Department. How can the nurse deal with this problem? Consider what can be done while care is given and what other measures another staff member could provide.

Exercise 2

Virtual Hospital Activity

60 minutes

You are an LPN who has been hired to work in the Pediatrics Unit. Because so many children come to the unit via the Emergency Department, your unit manager has assigned you to spend the day in the ED to learn about a child and his family's experiences there.

- Sign in to work at Pacific View Regional Hospital on the Pediatrics Floor for Period of Care 1. (*Note:* If you are already in the virtual hospital from a previous exercise, click on **Leave the Floor** and then on **Restart the Program** to get to the sign-in window.)
- From the Patient List, select Tommy Douglas (Room 302).
- Click on **Go to Nurses' Station**.
- Click on **Chart** and then on **302**.
- Click on and review the **Emergency Department** and **Physician's Orders** sections.

1. Review the circumstances behind Tommy Douglas' admission. Include such information as the nature of his injury and the people involved.

2. What are the priorities for care for Tommy Douglas?

3. Define *ventriculostomy*. What is the purpose of this procedure? (*Hint:* Try to identify key parts of the word that can help you with the definition. If necessary, you may refer to a medical dictionary).

4. A priority concern for Tommy Douglas is increased intracranial pressure (ICP). List the assessment areas that would indicate increasing ICP.

5. Which change in vital signs is indicative of increasing intracranial pressure?
   a. Decreased blood pressure
   b. Increased blood pressure
   c. Increased heart rate
   d. Increased respirations

- Return to the **Emergency Department** record in the chart. Check Tommy Douglas' admission vital signs.

6. Compare Tommy Douglas' vital signs to those of a healthy 6-year-old. How do they compare?

7. Do his vital signs reflect increased ICP?

8. You are shadowing a nurse who tells you that abnormal posturing is a sign of brain damage. Explain the differences between decerebrate and decorticate posturing.

- Click on and review the **History and Physical** tab for evidence of abnormal posturing.

9. Does Tommy Douglas manifest abnormal posturing at this point? (*Hint:* Changes may continue to develop as edema and bleeding in the brain increase.)

10. Why is Tommy Douglas receiving bolus infusions?

- Click the **Physician's Orders** tab and review the information given.

11. Review Tommy Douglas' initial medication orders (from admission on Tuesday through Wednesday morning). Below, match each medication with its corresponding use.

Medication	Use
_____ Cefazolin	a. Anticoagulant
_____ Dopamine	b. Electrolyte replacement
_____ Heparin	c. Maintenance of blood pressure
_____ Norepinephrine	d. Prevention of infection
_____ Sodium bicarbonate ($NaHCO_3$)	e. Treatment of ventricular fibrillation
_____ Vasopressin	f. Support of blood pressure

- Click on **Return to Nurses' Station**.
- Click on the **Drug** icon in the lower left corner of the screen.
- Review the medications ordered for Tommy Douglas.

12. You should note that $NaHCO_3$ is incompatible with both dopamine and norepinephrine. What does this mean in regard to administration?

13. Medications that are ordered STAT have to be given quickly. Generally, this means giving the

medication within a _____-minute time period.

You won't be administering critical care medications during your time in the Emergency Department. However, you do have the opportunity to practice medication administration in the virtual setting of Pacific View Regional Hospital. Select one of the medications that need to be administered during this period of care and complete the following steps to prepare and administer it.

- Click on **Return to Nurses' Station** and then on **Medication Room** at the bottom of the screen.
- Using the six rights, select, prepare, and administer the medication to be given. When you have finished the preparation, return to Tommy Douglas' room and administer the medication. (*Hint:* Although you should be getting more comfortable with the steps of preparing and administering medications, remember that you can refer to pages 24-28 and 35-39 in the **Getting Started** section if you need help.)
- To obtain feedback, click on **Leave the Floor**.
- Click on **Look at Your Preceptor's Evaluations** and then on **Medication Scorecard**.

14. Review the feedback on your Medication Scorecard. Are there any areas in which you need to make changes? If so, select another medication ordered for Tommy Douglas and practice the procedure again.

15. Reflect on your experience and comment on nursing responsibilities for medication administration in the Emergency Department.

- To return to the Pediatrics Floor, click on **Return to Evaluations**, **Return to Menu**, and **Restart the Program**.
- Sign in to work on the Pediatrics Floor for Period of Care 1.
- From the Patient List, select Tommy Douglas (Room 302).
- Click on **Go to Nurses' Station**.
- Click on **Chart** and then on **302**.
- Click on and review the **Physician's Orders** and **Nursing Admission**.

16. The physician has ordered a rate increase for norepinephrine. At what rate was the drug running? To what rate has it been increased?

17. The physician has ordered a rate increase for norepinephrine. What findings will indicate the medication dosage change has been effective?
    a. Heart rate will remain stable.
    b. Respiratory rate will increase.
    c. Blood pressure will increase.
    d. Blood pressure will decrease.

• Click on the **Emergency Department** tab and search the record for neurological assessment data.

18. Describe the Glasgow Coma Scale (GCS).

19. What significant neurological data did you find in Tommy Douglas' Emergency Department record?

20. Tommy Douglas is being stabilized in preparation for transfer to the Intensive Care Unit, and a cerebral perfusion scan is performed. What is the purpose of this test?

Exercise 3

Virtual Hospital Activity

20 minutes

1. It is determined that Tommy Douglas will not be going to the Intensive Care Unit as planned. He is instead being transferred to the Pediatric Unit for end-of-life care. Explain why you think this decision was made.

- Sign in to work at Pacific View Regional Hospital on the Pediatrics Floor for Period of Care 1. (*Note:* If you are already in the virtual hospital from a previous exercise, click on **Leave the Floor** and then on **Restart the Program** to get to the sign-in window.)
- From the Patient List, select Tommy Douglas (Room 302).
- Click on **Go to Nurses' Station** and then on **302** at the bottom of the screen.
- Click on **Patient Care** and complete a focused neurologic assessment of Tommy Douglas by clicking on **Neurologic** (yellow button) and then on the various body system subcategories (green buttons). Chart your findings in the EPR. (*Hint:* If you need help entering data in the EPR, refer to pages 15-16 in the **Getting Started** section of this workbook.)
- To obtain feedback, click **Leave the Floor** and then **Look at Your Preceptor's Evaluations**.
- Select **Examination Report** and review your evaluation.

2. Reflect on the completeness of your focused assessment of Tommy Douglas' neurologic status.

- To return to the Pediatrics Floor, click on **Return to Evaluations**, **Return to Menu**, and **Restart the Program**.
- Sign in to work on the Pediatrics Floor for Period of Care 1.
- From the Patient List, select Tommy Douglas (Room 302).
- Click on **Go to Nurses' Station** and then on **302** at the bottom of the screen.
- Click on **Patient Care** and then on **Nurse-Client Interactions**.
- Select and view the video titled **0730: Assessment—Neurological**. (*Note:* Check the virtual clock to see whether enough time has elapsed. You can use the fast-forward feature to advance the time by 2-minute intervals if the video is not yet available. Then click again on **Patient Care** and **Nurse-Client Interactions** to refresh the screen.)

3. What was Tommy Douglas' GCS score at this time?

4. Consider how well the nurse explained the purpose and meaning of the GCS to Tommy Douglas' parents. Do you think the parents found support during this interaction? What, if anything, would you have done differently?

- Click again on **Patient Care** and then on **Nurse-Client Interactions**.
- Select and view the video titled **0745: Intervention—Airway**. (*Note:* Check the virtual clock to see whether enough time has elapsed. You can use the fast-forward feature to advance the time by 2-minute intervals if the video is not yet available. Then click again on **Patient Care** and **Nurse-Client Interactions** to refresh the screen.)

5. Tommy Douglas is on a ventilator. What is a ventilator used for? How would you expect Tommy Douglas' ventilator to be set?

6. How would you explain to Tommy Douglas' parents what the ventilator is doing?

- Once again, click on **Patient Care** and then on **Nurse-Client Interactions**.
- Select and view the video titled **0800: Intervention—Stabilizing Blood Pressure**. (*Note:* Check the virtual clock to see whether enough time has elapsed. You can use the fast-forward feature to advance the time by 2-minute intervals if the video is not yet available. Then click again on **Patient Care** and **Nurse-Client Interactions** to refresh the screen.)

7. Tommy Douglas' blood pressure is low. Explain why fluids help to maintain blood pressure.

Tommy Douglas will be receiving end-of-life care. Continue to the next lesson to learn about nursing care for the parents and family of a child who is dying.

Providing Support for Families Experiencing the Loss of a Child

Reading Assignment: The Child with a Sensory or Neurological Condition (Chapter 23)
The Child with a Condition of the Blood, Blood-Forming Organs, or Lymphatic System (Chapter 27)

Patient: Tommy Douglas, Pediatrics Floor, Room 302

Objectives:

1. Explore the range of reactions that may occur when parents are told there is no hope of saving their child's life.
2. Discuss the role of hospital ethics committees.
3. Discuss nursing responsibilities associated with organ donation.
4. Discuss the concept of "allowing" a child to die.
5. Identify strategies to support parents and other children as a child dies.

In this lesson you will explore circumstances that may occur in hospital settings around a traumatic event resulting in certainty of death. Care for parents and other family members is the major focus during this time of hospice care. You will continue to work with the family of 6-year-old Tommy Douglas as he dies.

Exercise 1

Writing Activity

20 minutes

"Allowing" a child to die is a very difficult concept. Parents go through several stages of emotion as their child dies.

1. Discuss what parents go through when their child experiences a life-threatening injury or illness that then becomes terminal.

2. Parents frequently need to talk about what is happening while their child is dying. Why?

3. What signs are present during the dying process that are indicative of imminent death?

4. Assume that you enter the room and find parents sobbing as they sit with their dying child. Does this mean you have not been effective with your teaching and care? What can you do for these parents?

5. How might you guide parents at the time of death? (*Hint:* Remember that allowing a child to die is tremendously difficult for parents and is often perceived as out of the order of natural events.)

6. What are your thoughts about how you would provide care for the family members after the death of the child?

7. Discuss ways that nurses who care for dying children cope with their own grief.

Exercise 2

Virtual Hospital Activity

45 minutes

- Sign in to work at Pacific View Regional Hospital on the Pediatrics Floor for Period of Care 2. (*Note:* If you are already in the virtual hospital from a previous exercise, click on **Leave the Floor** and then on **Restart the Program** to get to the sign-in window.)
- From the Patient List, select Tommy Douglas (Room 302).
- Click on **Go to Nurses' Station** and then on **302** at the bottom of the screen.
- Click on **Patient Care** and then on **Nurse-Client Interactions**.
- Select and view the video titled **1115: The Family (Care) Conference**. (*Note:* Check the virtual clock to see whether enough time has elapsed. You can use the fast-forward feature to advance the time by 2-minute intervals if the video is not yet available. Then click again on **Patient Care** and **Nurse-Client Interactions** to refresh the screen.)

1. Tommy Douglas has been certified as "brain dead," and a family conference has been arranged to inform his parents that he will not be helped by further intervention. Who are the usual participants in such a conference? What does each person bring to the discussion?

2. What intervention can the nurse provide to the parents after the family conference?

3. What if Tommy Douglas' parents say that they want him to live "at all costs"? How would you feel about this?

4. Discuss how your response to the previous question might affect your care for Tommy Douglas' parents.

- Again, click on **Patient Care** and then on **Nurse-Client Interactions**.
- Select and view the video titled **1130: Decision—Organ Donation**. (*Note:* Check the virtual clock to see whether enough time has elapsed. You can use the fast-forward feature to advance the time by 2-minute intervals if the video is not yet available. Then click again on **Patient Care** and **Nurse-Client Interactions** to refresh the screen.)

5. Tommy Douglas' parents have agreed to organ donation. Does this provide evidence of progression with anticipatory grieving?

6. Visit the website for United Network for Organ Sharing (*www.unos.org*) and discuss the criteria for donation and management of a potential donor.

- Click on **Chart** and then on **302**.
- Click on the **Physician's Orders** tab and review.

7. Discuss the type of care that is being provided for Tommy Douglas during this time.

8. Tommy Douglas is to receive hospice care. Compare palliative and hospice care. (*Hint:* You may want to refer to your medical dictionary.)

Let's check in on Tommy Douglas' family a little later in the day.

- Click on **Return to Nurses' Station**.
- Click on **Leave the Floor** and then on **Restart the Program**.
- Sign in to work on the Pediatrics Floor for Period of Care 3.
- From the Patient List, select Tommy Douglas (Room 302).
- Click on **Go to Nurses' Station** and then on **302** at the bottom of the screen.
- Click on **Patient Care** and then on **Nurse-Client Interactions**.
- Select and view the video titled **1500: Nurse—Family Communication**. (*Note:* Check the virtual clock to see whether enough time has elapsed. You can use the fast-forward feature to advance the time by 2-minute intervals if the video is not yet available. Then click again on **Patient Care** and **Nurse-Client Interactions** to refresh the screen.)

9. Evaluate the nurse's approach to dealing with a family in crisis. Did the nurse demonstrate empathy? If so, how?

10. Is the nurse's body language congruent with his verbal communication?

11. Present an alternative to the nurse's approach if you believe it is indicated.

You need to learn more about Tommy Douglas' family, especially whether or not he has siblings.

- Click on **Chart** and then on **302**.
- Click on **History and Physical** and review Tommy Douglas' family configuration.

12. Tommy Douglas has a brother who is 8 years old. Which description best expresses his likely understanding of death and dying?
    a. Recognizes death as final
    b. Has a grasp of the abstract concept of death
    c. May have feeling of self-responsibility for sibling's death
    d. May view death as temporary

13. When interacting with Tommy Douglas' 4-year-old sister, which approach will be most effective?
    a. Encouraging the parents to allow the child to participate in the funeral
    b. Encouraging communication and discussion
    c. Offering reassurance to the child
    d. Recognizing the child is primarily responding to the anxiety and sadness being expressed by the parents

- Click on the **Nursing Admission** tab and review the information given.
- Click on **Return to Room 302**.
- Click on **Patient Care** and then on **Nurse-Client Interactions**.
- Select and view the video titled **1515: The Grieving Family**. (*Note:* Check the virtual clock to see whether enough time has elapsed. You can use the fast-forward feature to advance the time by 2-minute intervals if the video is not yet available. Then click again on **Patient Care** and **Nurse-Client Interactions** to refresh the screen.)

14. How are siblings of a dying child likely to view death?

15. _____ The parents of a child who has died have a higher rate of divorce. (True or False)

16. For parents who have lost a child, what anticipatory guidance could you offer for dealing with other children in their family?

Notes:

Notes:

Notes:

Notes:

Notes:

Notes:

Notes:

Notes: